T0245212

Handbook of Tuberculosis

Jacques H. Grosset
Richard E. Chaisson
Editors

Handbook of
Tuberculosis

 Adis

Editors

Jacques H. Grosset
Johns Hopkins Center for TB
Research
Baltimore, Maryland, USA

Richard E. Chaisson
Johns Hopkins Center for TB
Research
Baltimore, Maryland, USA

ISBN 978-3-319-26271-0   ISBN 978-3-319-26273-4   (eBook)
DOI 10.1007/978-3-319-26273-4

Library of Congress Control Number: 2017930127

Printed on acid-free paper

This Adis imprint is published by Springer Nature
The registered company is Springer International Publishing AG
The registered company address is: Gewerbestrasse 11, 6330 Cham, Switzerland

Abbreviations

ADA	Adenosine deaminase activity
AFB	Acid fast bacilli
AIDS	Acquired immune deficiency Syndrome
ALT	Alanine aminotransferase (formerly SGPT)
ART	Antiretroviral therapy
AST	Aspartate aminotransferase (formerly SGOT)
BCG	Bacillus Calmette Guérin
CD4	T-helper cells or T4 cells
CDC	Center for Disease Control
CFP-10	Culture filtrate protein 10
CNS	Central nervous system
CRISPR	Clustered regularly interspaced short palindromic repeats
CSF	Cerebrospinal fluid
CT	Computerized tomography
DNA	Deoxyribonucleic acid
DOT	Directly observed therapy
DTH	Delayed-type hypersensitivity
EBA	Early bactericidal activity
EPTB	Extrapulmonary tuberculosis
ESAT-6	The 6 kDa early secretory antigenic Target
GC	Guanine cytosine
HAART	Highly active antiretroviral therapy
HIV	Human immunodeficiency virus
IFN-γ	Interferon-gamma

IGRA	Interferon-gamma release assay
IL-12	Interleukin 12
INH	Isoniazid
IPT	Isoniazid preventive therapy
IRIS	Immune reconstitution inflammatory syndrome
IS6110	Insertion sequence 6110
LMIC	Low and middle income countries
LTBI	Latent tuberculosis infection
MDR	Multidrug-resistant
MDR-TB	Multidrug-resistant tuberculosis
MIC	Minimum inhibitory concentration
MRI	Magnetic resonance imaging
MTB	Mycobacterium tuberculosis
NAA	Nucleic acid amplification
NAAT	Nucleic acid amplification testing
NRTI	Nucleoside reverse transcriptase inhibitors
PCR	Polymerase chain reaction
PLWHA	Persons living with HIV and/or AIDS
POA	Pyrazinoic acid
PZA	Pyrazinamide
QFT-GIT	QuantiFERON-TB In Tube
RIF	Ripampin/rifampicin
RNA	Ribonucleic acid
SGOT	Serum glutamic oxaloacetic transaminase
SGPT	Serum glutamic pyruvic transaminase
TB	Tuberculosis
TBM	TB meningitis
TNF-α	Tumor necrosis factor α
TST	Tuberculin skin test
WHO	World Health Organization
XDR-TB	Extensively drug-resistant tuberculosis
Xpert MTB/RIF	Automated NAAT diagnostic test to identify MTB DNA and resistance to RIF

Contents

Biography

Editors

Jacques H. Grosset, M.D., is a Professor of Medicine at the Center for TB Research, Division of Infectious Diseases, Department of Medicine, Johns Hopkins University School of Medicine. He was trained in medicine at the Lille University, Lille, France, and in microbiology and immunology at the Pasteur Institute, Paris, France, under the mentorship of George Canetti. His main area of research is the chemotherapy of mycobacterial infections, including tuberculosis, leprosy, M. avium infection in the immune deficient host and M. ulcerans infection (Buruli ulcer). He currently focuses his efforts on the shortening of treatment duration and prevention of drug resistance.

Richard E. Chaisson, M.D., is a Professor of Medicine, Epidemiology, and International Health at Johns Hopkins University in Baltimore, USA. He received his B.S. and M.D. degrees from the University of Massachusetts and was an intern, resident, and fellow at the University of California, San Francisco, USA, where he was also Assistant Professor of Medicine. From 1988 to 1998, he was Director of the Johns Hopkins AIDS Service, and he co-founded the Johns Hopkins HIV Clinic cohort, an observational study that has been the source of more than 130 scientific publications on the outcomes of HIV disease and its treatment. Dr. Chaisson is currently Director of the Johns Hopkins Center for Tuberculosis

Research, a multidisciplinary center with more than $60 million in grants for the study of tuberculosis from bench to bedside. Dr. Chaisson's research interests focus on tuberculosis and HIV infection, including global epidemiology, clinical trials, diagnostics, and public health interventions. He is currently principal investigator of 11 research grants, and is Director of the Consortium to Respond Effectively to the AIDS/TB Epidemic (CREATE), an international research consortium funded by the Bill and Melinda Gates Foundation to assess the impact of novel strategies for controlling HIV-related tuberculosis. He has published over 300 scientific papers and book chapters.

Contributors

William Bishai, M.D., Ph.D., is a Professor of Medicine in the Division of Infectious Diseases and Co-Director of the Center for TB Research at the Johns Hopkins School of Medicine. He was trained in medicine and microbiology at Harvard Medical School, Boston MA, USA, and in infectious diseases at the Johns Hopkins Hospital, Baltimore, MD, USA. His main areas of research include tuberculosis mechanisms of pathogenesis and development of tools to combat TB including drugs, diagnostics, and vaccines. He currently serves on the editorial boards and NIH review panels. His main clinical activity is with the inpatient infectious disease service at Johns Hopkins Hospital.

Natasha Chida, M.D., MSPH, is a clinical fellow in the Division of Infectious Diseases, Johns Hopkins University School of Medicine. She was trained in medicine and public health at the University of Miami Miller School of Medicine, completed internal medicine residency and a chief residency at Jackson Memorial Hospital/the University of Miami Miller School of Medicine, and will complete her infectious disease fellowship at Johns Hopkins University. Her primary area of research involves how to best deliver graduate medical education in both the United States and the global arena. She is also interested in developing educational content for medical professionals in the United States and in resource-limited settings. Her clinical interests are focused in HIV and TB care.

Kelly E. Dooley, M.D., Ph.D., MPH, is an Associate Professor of Medicine, Pharmacology and Molecular Sciences at the Johns Hopkins University School of Medicine. She was trained in medicine at Duke University and public health at University of North Carolina Chapel Hill. She completed Internal Medicine and Infectious Diseases training at Johns Hopkins, as well as a fellowship in Clinical Pharmacology and Ph.D. at the School of Public Health. Her research interests include optimization of treatment of drug-sensitive and drug-resistant TB, including for special populations such as children and pregnant women; HIV-TB co-treatment; and pharmacology of anti-TB drugs.

Susan E. Dorman, M.D., is Professor of Medicine at Johns Hopkins University School of Medicine, Baltimore, Maryland, USA. She received her medical degree from Duke University School of Medicine, and subsequently trained in internal medicine at the Brigham and Women's Hospital in Boston, Massachusetts, and in infectious diseases at the National Institutes of Health, Bethesda, Maryland. The focus of her research is the identification of new diagnostic and treatment approaches for tuberculosis. She provides clinical care at the Johns Hopkins Hospital and the Baltimore Health Department Eastern Chest Clinic.

David Dowdy, M.D., ScM, Ph.D., is an Associate Professor of Epidemiology at the Johns Hopkins Bloomberg School of Public Health. He received his B.S. in chemistry from Duke University, North Carolina, USA, and his ScM and Ph.D. in epidemiology as well as M.D. from Johns Hopkins University, Maryland, USA. He completed residency training in internal medicine at the University of California, San Francisco,

USA. His research centers on case-finding and diagnosis of tuberculosis (including HIV-associated and drug-resistant tuberculosis), with a particular interest in the synthesis of implementation science, transmission modeling, and economic evaluation. He serves on the steering committee for the TB Modeling and Analysis Consortium and has published over 100 peer-reviewed articles in the scientific literature. He practices general internal medicine in urban East Baltimore.

Noton K. Dutta, Ph.D., is a Research Associate of Medicine at the Johns Hopkins University School of Medicine. Dr. Dutta obtained his Ph.D. from Jadavpur University, India, and did postdoctoral research at Seoul National University, South Korea, and Tulane University, USA. He completed his senior postdoctoral fellowship in Dr. Karakousis' laboratory and joined the faculty in 2015. Dr. Dutta has significant expertise in microbiology, molecular biology, and animal models of TB infection.

His research focuses on characterizing the efficacy of novel drugs and drug combinations against M. tuberculosis in murine and guinea pig models, with the goal of shortening the duration of TB chemotherapy. He is using multidisciplinary techniques, including computational modeling and high-throughput genetic screens in various animal models, including nonhuman primates, in order to elucidate M. tuberculosis essential pathways involved in latency and reactivation, as well as detection of TB biomarkers in people with HIV infection. He has published over 60 peer-reviewed papers on relevant topics.

Jonathan Golub, Ph.D., is an Associate Professor of Medicine, Epidemiology and International Health at the Johns Hopkins University School of Medicine and the Johns Hopkins Bloomberg School of Public Health, Maryland, USA. He received his BA in Biology and History from the State University of New York at Binghamton, New York, USA, his MPH in Epidemiology from Columbia University Mailman School of Public Health, New York, USA, and his Ph.D. in

Epidemiology from Johns Hopkins Bloomberg School of Public Health. His research focuses on the epidemiology of TB in South Africa, India, Brazil, and the USA, with specific focus on the drivers of TB in these settings. He teaches the "Epidemiologic Basis for TB Control" at the Bloomberg School of Public Health and through several training grants has mentored over 100 researchers in Brazil, South Africa, and India. He has published over 90 peer-reviewed articles in the scientific literature.

Amita Gupta, M.D., MPH, is an Associate Professor of Medicine and International Health at Johns Hopkins University School of Medicine and Bloomberg School of Public Health, Baltimore, Maryland, USA. She received her medical degree from Harvard Medical School, and subsequently trained in internal medicine at San Francisco General Hospital, University of California, San Francisco; in Epidemic Intelligence Service at US Centers for Disease Control and Prevention; and in infectious diseases and clinical epidemiology at Johns Hopkins University. The focus of her research is the prevention and treatment of TB among adults (including pregnant women) and children residing in low and middle income countries with focus on India. She provides clinical care at the Johns Hopkins Hospital.

Sanjay Jain, M.D., is an Associate Professor of Pediatrics and International Health at the Johns Hopkins Children's Center. He was trained in medicine at the All India Institute of Medical Sciences, New Delhi. He did his internship at Penn State Children's Hospital, Pediatric residency at Floating Hospital for Children (Tufts), and a fellowship in Pediatric Infectious Diseases at the Johns Hopkins Hospitals. His main areas of research include development of novel imaging technologies for bacterial infections, pediatric tuberculosis (TB), and CNS TB.

Petros C. Karakousis, M.D., is an Associate Professor of Medicine at the Johns Hopkins University School of Medicine.

His research is primarily focused on understanding the molecular basis of *Mycobacterium tuberculosis* persistence and reactivation. His laboratory is also involved in the pre-clinical testing of novel antimicrobial drugs and host-directed therapy for TB in clinically relevant animal models, as well as the development of novel molecular assays for the rapid diagnosis of latent TB infection and active TB disease, and for the detection of drug resistance. Dr. Karakousis received his undergraduate degree from the Johns Hopkins University and his medical degree from Washington University School of Medicine in St. Louis. He completed residency training in Internal Medicine at the Hospital of the University of Pennsylvania and fellowship training in Infectious Diseases at Johns Hopkins University School of Medicine. Dr. Karakousis is a Fellow of the Infectious Diseases Society of America and a member of the Editorial Board of *Journal of Infectious Diseases* and *PLoS One*.

Gyanu Lamichhane, Ph.D., is an Associate Professor in the Division of Infectious Diseases, Department of Medicine, Johns Hopkins University School of Medicine. Trained in cellular and molecular medicine, he wrote thesis in genes and targets essential for viability and growth of *Mycobacterium tuberculosis*. His current research focuses on identification and characterization of essential proteins of peptidoglycan biosynthesis and development of new antibacterials that work by interfering with peptidoglycan biosynthesis. Investigating fundamental aspects of microbial life and exploiting the findings to develop clinically useful tools are the philosophical foundations of his efforts.

Yukari C. Manabe, M.D., is the Associate Director of Global Health Research and Innovation within the Johns Hopkins Center for Global Health, a Professor of Medicine, International Health, and Molecular Microbiology and Immunology. She began her faculty career as a basic science researcher studying the molecular and immune-pathogenesis of tuberculosis (TB) in animal models. From 2007 until 2012, she was seconded from JHU to build research capacity at the Infectious Diseases Institute in Kampala, Uganda, as the Head of Research. Her research focuses on HIV and TB-HIV co-infection in sub-Saharan Africa and on the validation and introduction of frugal innovation in infectious disease diagnostics to improve diagnostic certainty in resource-limited settings. Dr. Manabe obtained her undergraduate degree from Yale University and her M.D. from Columbia University College of Physicians and Surgeons. She joined the Johns Hopkins School of Medicine faculty in 1999 after completing her residency in internal medicine and fellowship in Infectious Diseases at Johns Hopkins Hospital.

Nicole Salazar-Austin, M.D., is a clinical fellow in pediatric infectious disease at the Johns Hopkins University School of Medicine. She was trained in medicine at Harvard Medical School, Boston, USA, and in pediatrics at the Children's Hospital of Philadelphia, Philadelphia, USA. Her main areas of research include prevention of pediatric tuberculosis and optimization of health care delivery in the developing world.

Maunank Shah, M.D., Ph.D., is an Assistant Professor in the Division of Infectious Diseases, Center for TB Research, Johns Hopkins University School of Medicine. He was trained in medicine at University of California—San Francisco, completed internal medicine residency at Emory University, and completed infectious disease fellowship and a Ph.D. in clinical investigation at Johns Hopkins University. His primary areas of research include evaluation of TB diagnostics, epidemiologic and economic modeling of HIV and TB interventions, and usage of mobile health technologies to improve treatment adherence. He is the Medical Director for the Baltimore City Health Dept TB program, serves as Associate Editor for OFID, an IDSA journal, and is the Co-Director for the Microbiology/Infectious Diseases curriculum at Johns Hopkins School of Medicine.

Chapter 1
Overview of Tuberculosis

Richard E. Chaisson and William R. Bishai

1.1 History

Tuberculosis has plagued mankind for millennia, causing disease, deformity, and death since prehistoric times. Mummies from ancient civilizations have been found to have evidence of tuberculosis, and the organism has been amplified from archeological relics from more than 5000 years ago [1]. While pulmonary tuberculosis is and most likely always has been the most common form of the disease, extrapulmonary forms of tuberculosis have a prominent place in history. Scrofula, tuberculosis of the cervical lymph nodes, was said to have been cured by the royal touch of kings, from King Clovis of France in the fifth century to Edward the Confessor, King of England in the eleventh century, and subsequently. Pott's disease, tuberculosis of the spine which can cause grave

R.E. Chaisson (✉)
Departments of Medicine, Epidemiology, and International Health, Johns Hopkins University, Baltimore, MD, USA
e-mail: rchaiss@jhmi.edu

W.R. Bishai
Department of Medicine, Division of Infectious Diseases, JHU School of Medicine,
CRB2 Room 108 / 1550 Orleans St, 20287 Baltimore, MD, USA
e-mail: wbishai1@jhmi.edu

J.H. Grosset, R.E. Chaisson (eds.), *Handbook of Tuberculosis*,
DOI 10.1007/978-3-319-26273-4_1,
© Springer International Publishing Switzerland 2017

deformity, is the possible cause of the gibbus affliction of Quasimodo, the famed Hunchback of Notre Dame. Tuberculosis was the actual cause of death for many famous literary figures, from the Bronte sisters to Robert Louis Stephenson to Stephen Crane.

Tuberculosis emerged as an epidemic disease in Europe in the Middle Ages and became a leading cause of death for centuries to follow. The most common and lethal form of the disease was and remains pulmonary disease, and the term "consumption" was applied to those with the wasting illness accompanied by severe respiratory symptoms, sputum production, hemoptysis, and eventually death. In his classic *The Life and Death of Mr. Badman* (1680), John Bunyan wrote, "Yet the captain of all these men of death that came against him to take him away, was the consumption, for it was that that brought him down to the grave" [2]. From the 1600s through the late 1800s, tuberculosis caused between 20 and 30 % of all deaths in London and similar proportions throughout England, Wales, Scotland, and the USA [3]. While the disease was romanticized in opera, painting, poetry, and literature, the grim reality of its ruthless toll on humanity was staggering.

In the twentieth century, tuberculosis continued to cause massive suffering and death, but rates of the disease fell for a number of decades as other causes of death, war, famine, influenza, and smallpox, grew more fearsome. The decline in tuberculosis incidence and mortality in the decades before the development of effective treatment has been widely credited to socioeconomic advances, with improved nutrition, better housing with more sunlight and better ventilation, and an overall increase in social welfare listed as possible causes of the waning of the epidemic [4]. In addition, the rise of tuberculosis sanatoria, which isolated infectious patients in remote locations where much time was spent outdoors where ultraviolet light was abundant, has also been cited as a contributing factor. An alternative hypothesis is that coevolution of the organism and its host resulted in more effective immunity in humans, as natural selection killed many with poor defenses, and possibly a less virulent organism that lived in better symbiosis with its obligate vector [5]. The discovery of the tubercle bacillus by Robert Koch in 1882 was the beginning of a century of scientific triumph over the disease. Koch's momentous announcement of a microbial cause of *phthisis*, or consumption, was followed by the isolation of tuberculin, thought by Koch to be therapeutic against the disease but ultimately playing an important diagnostic role; the development of a live, attenuated vaccine, the bacille Calmette-Guérin, or BCG; the discovery of streptomycin by Schatz, Bugie, and Waksman; and the creation of a potent armamentarium of antimicrobial agents effect against this once untreatable and highly lethal infection [6]. By the 1980s, 100 years after Koch's breakthrough, tuberculosis could be treated and cured in virtually all patients who were treated with an oral regimen of drugs taken for as little as 6 months [7]. In addition, the use of oral isoniazid had been shown to be highly effective in preventing tuberculosis in high-risk populations [8].

The triumph of science over disease was celebrated with two Nobel Prizes, to Koch and Waksman,[1] resulted in the closure of tuberculosis sanatoria around the globe, granted life to those formerly condemned, and had enormous socioeconomic benefit. With diagnostics, effective treatment, preventive therapy, and a vaccine in hand, science moved on to other priorities and problems, and tuberculosis research was left in a vacuum. Funding for tuberculosis research in the USA fell dramatically between 1962 and 1972, to virtually nil [9].

While scientists, physicians, public health officials, and the public were toasting the end of tuberculosis, the disease was busy continuing its deadly assault on humanity. Trends in tuberculosis incidence and death experienced an accelerated decline in the USA, UK, Europe, and other developed areas, but the disease continued to inflict heavy casualties in more resource poor nations in Africa, Asia, and Latin America. A common and credible belief is that the failure to control tuberculosis in these parts of the world was the result of weak

[1] A third Nobel Prize to Niels Finsen in 1903 for phototherapy of cutaneous tuberculosis was clearly an error.

health systems that were unable to deliver the miraculous technological advances brought forth by researchers over the previous century. Countering this hypothesis are the limitations of the tools available for tuberculosis control in the latter part of the twentieth century, however. The BCG vaccine became and remains the most widely used vaccine in the world (and in history), yet there is little evidence that it has had an impact on the tuberculosis epidemic as it does not appear to protect against pulmonary tuberculosis in adults, who are the primary vectors of infection. The most widely used diagnostic test for tuberculosis, the sputum acid-fast bacilli (AFB) smear, is notoriously insensitive, missing 50 % or more pulmonary cases. The miracle of oral, outpatient tuberculosis treatment was undercut by poor adherence for the full 6–9 months required to cure the disease, resulting in treatment failure and emergence of drug resistance.

Against this backdrop of the frailty of the tools for global tuberculosis control, two critically important epidemiologic developments arose which have dramatically altered the course of the disease over the past three decades. The emergence of HIV has had a catastrophic impact on tuberculosis worldwide, fueling an explosive rise in tuberculosis incidence in people living with HIV everywhere and stunning increases in national tuberculosis incidence rates in sub-Saharan Africa, where two-thirds of people with HIV infection live [10]. The second major epidemiologic shift over the past several decades has been the emergence of drug-resistant tuberculosis [11]. Multidrug-resistant (MDR) tuberculosis and now extensively drug-resistant (XDR) tuberculosis now account for about 5 % of all cases worldwide and pose substantial challenges in diagnosis and treatment.

1.2   Global Impact

The global impact of tuberculosis remains enormous. In 2015, tuberculosis was declared the leading cause of death by an infection worldwide, surpassing HIV infection [12]. Approximately

1.5 million individuals were estimated to have died of tuberculosis the previous year, compared with 1.2 million dying with HIV. Of note, about 400,000 people died with both HIV *and* tuberculosis, and these deaths are attributed to HIV under international disease classification coding. Nevertheless, the burden of suffering and death caused by tuberculosis is massive. The WHO estimates almost 10 million new cases occurred in 2014, and one-third of these were not properly diagnosed and treated. Recent estimates show that about 10 % of tuberculosis cases globally are in children <15 years old or almost 1 million cases of pediatric tuberculosis in 2010 [13]. And MDR tuberculosis occurred in an estimated 450,000 individuals in 2014 [12].

The distribution of tuberculosis worldwide disproportionately affects Africa, Asia, and Eastern Europe, while Western Europe, the USA and Canada, and Oceania experience far lower rates of disease. Figure 1.1 shows WHO estimates of tuberculosis incidence rates per 100,000 population by country [12]. The highest case rates are generally in sub-Saharan Africa, where HIV infection has spurred large increases in incidence over the past 25 years. Countries such as Botswana, South Africa, Swaziland, and Lesotho have rates of tuberculosis that are >500/100,000 or more than 150-fold greater than the USA. The countries of South Asia and the Western Pacific have considerably lower incidence rates but extremely large populations, and India and China together account for almost 40 % of global cases of tuberculosis. For the past 20 years, the WHO has focused attention on the 22 so-called high-burden countries, nations which account for 80 % of the global tuberculosis burden. This list of countries includes India and China, but also countries with smaller populations but higher incidence rates, such as South Africa, Nigeria, and Tanzania. Under the new "End TB" strategy developed by the WHO, the list of high-burden countries has expanded to 30 and is categorized into nations with high overall rates of tuberculosis, high rates of tuberculosis and HIV, and high rates of MDR tuberculosis [12]. These grouping highlight the specific types of challenges faced in addressing specific epidemiologic aspects of the disease at a national level.

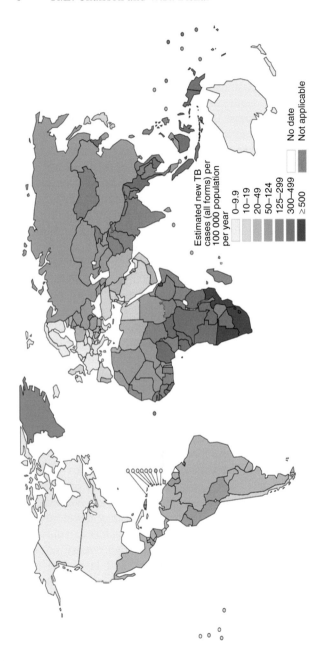

Fig. 1.1 Global incidence of tuberculosis by country (Reproduced with permission from Global Tuberculosis Report 2015 [12], ©World Health Organization 2015. All rights reserved)

Estimated new TB cases (all forms) per 100 000 population per year

0–9.9
10–19
20–49
50–124
125–299
300–499
≥500

No date

Not applicable

MDR tuberculosis is found worldwide, but the countries of Eastern Europe have especially high rates, and many cases are reported in South Africa, India, China, and Peru. MDR tuberculosis is historically a man-made phenomenon, produced by improper prescription of or adherence to treatment. Drug resistance generally appeared in patients whose treatment was mismanaged, interrupted, or irregular, and selection of resistant mutants was facilitated. The prevalence of MDR tuberculosis in patients with previous treatment has been and remains substantially higher than in patients with no previous exposure to antituberculosis therapy. However, as the prevalence of MDR tuberculosis has increased over the past decade, drug-resistant strains are increasingly transmitted, and a growing number of cases of MDR tuberculosis are appearing in patients with a first episode of disease [13]. This dramatic change in the epidemiology of MDR tuberculosis requires a shift in strategies for combating resistant disease. As a consequence, drug susceptibility testing of all tuberculosis patients, especially those in higher prevalence settings, is essential to ensure rapid identification of resistance and initiation of appropriate treatment.

A noteworthy aspect of the impact of tuberculosis and its fellow infectious killers – HIV, malaria, and bacterial pneumonia – is that they cause the most suffering and loss of life in the young, young adults in the case of tuberculosis and HIV and children in the case of malaria and bacterial pneumonia. The so-called noncommunicable diseases, cardiovascular disease, cancer, diabetes, and chronic lung disease, tend to strike older individuals and while contributing to a large number of deaths worldwide have a less severe socioeconomic cost. The premature loss of life – with its attendant impacts on family life, social structure, community institutions, and economic productivity of nations – caused by tuberculosis has a disproportionate impact in the high-burden countries. The WHO estimates that 52 % of all years of life lost (premature mortality) worldwide is due to infectious diseases, while only 34 % is from the noncommunicable diseases [12]. (The remaining 14 % is due to trauma.) Hence, investment in measures to diagnose, treat, and prevent tuberculosis has the potential to reap important socioeconomic benefits on top of the health benefits of controlling the disease.

1.3   Etiology

Tuberculosis is caused by the gram-positive, acid-fast bacillus, *Mycobacterium tuberculosis* and closely related species including *M. africanum* and *M. bovis*. While there are hundreds of other species within the genus *Mycobacterium*, most are environmental saprophytic species which are either non-pathogens (e.g., *M. smegmatis*) or opportunistic pathogens (e.g., *M. avium*, *M. chelonae*). *M. tuberculosis*, *M. africanum*, and *M. bovis* are pathogens capable of creating disease in fully immunocompetent individuals. The basis for this innate pathogenicity is under intense study, and it is clear that *M. tuberculosis* harbors unique virulence factors for subverting host immunity and creating disease.

Robert Koch first identified *M. tuberculosis* as the causative agent of tuberculosis in 1882 by demonstrating the presence of "acid-fast" bacilli (bacterial forms that retained dye despite the use of acid-alcohol destaining) in tuberculous tissues. Soon thereafter the microbe was grown in simple broth cultures. An unusual feature of *M. tuberculosis* is its slow doubling time of ~24 h. Consequently, it takes several weeks for cultures to show evidence of growth. The basis for the slow growth of *M. tuberculosis* and related mycobacteria remains uncertain.

In addition to slow growth, mycobacteria are unusual for their possession of a distinctive cell envelope. A characteristic feature of the envelope is the presence of mycolic acids – 60–90 carbon in length – which are covalently attached to the peptidoglycan layer of the envelope. The mycolic acids of mycobacteria are responsible for their characteristic acid-fastness and also are responsible for the characteristic clumping of organisms seen microscopically. Importantly, having mycolic acids is essential for mycobacterial viability. Several key antituberculous drugs act by inhibiting either the synthesis of mycolic acids themselves or of the support structure which links them to the microbial cell wall [14].

The genome of *M. tuberculosis* was first elucidated in 1998, and since then several thousands of different isolates of the species have also been subjected to genome sequencing. The genome is a single circular chromosome of 4.4 million base pairs encoding 3959 genes and is 66 % GC [15]. The genome has several repetitive elements including transposable elements such as IS6110 as well as a CRISPR system with variable regions flanked by invariant spacers, and these elements have been exploited for strain typing. More recently, whole genome sequencing has been used to classify isolates from disease outbreaks. The genomic studies reveal that *M. tuberculosis* has a slow rate of mutation acquisition, about 0.7 base variations per year over time during spread through human populations [16]. Additionally, genomics has permitted the identification of seven major lineages of *M. tuberculosis*; these lineages are defined by their genetic proximity to most recent common ancestor strains. The "species" *M. bovis* and *M. africanum* are actually sub-elements of the larger phylogeny of *M. tuberculosis* with *M. bovis* being a branch of lineage 6 and *M. africanum* being found in both lineages 5 and 6 [17]. While it has long been hypothesized that certain subtypes of *M. tuberculosis* might be more pathogenic for humans or be predisposed to causing certain variations of the disease, this has yet to be shown definitively, and it is clear that all seven lineages are capable of causing human TB.

Finally, while tuberculosis is caused by the bacterium, *M. tuberculosis*, it is also clear that human genetics plays an important role in the etiology of TB. Families which have high susceptibility to TB have been identified and characterized, and these studies have identified rare hereditary defects in the IL12-interferon-gamma axis of cell-mediated immunity [18]. However, beyond these rare hereditary defects, there may be more commonplace host genetic backgrounds which predispose to resistance or susceptibility. Aboriginal populations including the Inuits of North America and certain tribes in the Amazonian rainforest were more susceptible to tuberculosis than the Caucasian travelers who first contacted them and exposed them to TB for the first time [19]. During an accidental exposure, known as the Lubeck disaster, during which 240 infants under the age of 10 days were mistakenly inoculated with the same amount of virulent *M. tuberculosis* instead of the intended vaccine strain, about 70 % of the children did not progress to fatal disease [20]. The immunogenetics of human susceptibility to TB is a topic under considerable study.

1.4   Epidemiology

The natural history of tuberculosis begins with infection of a host, establishment of latent or subclinical infection, and progression to active disease, which occurs in only a small proportion of those infected [21]. The organism is transmitted by the airborne route when individuals with active respiratory tract infections expel bacilli into the environment. Humans are both the obligate host and vector of *M. tuberculosis*, and no other reservoirs of infection exist. *M. bovis* causes disease in cattle and other mammals that have had contact with diseased animals, such as water buffalo, lions, giraffes, and badgers; transmission to humans can occur through contaminated dairy products, but this is not an epidemiologically important pathway.

Figure 1.2 is a schematic drawing of the population dynamics of tuberculosis, illustrating the chain of transmission, with latent infections becoming active disease resulting in infection of the uninfected/susceptible, and new infections either progressing to early disease or latent infection which can reactivate in the future [22]. Control measures are also shown: diagnosis and treatment of active tuberculosis diseases halt further transmission, an effective vaccine would protect the uninfected, and treatment of latent tuberculosis prevents transmissible forms of the disease from occurring at all. Additional measures to control disease at the population

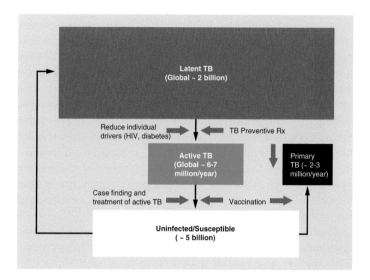

Fig. 1.2 Population dynamics of global tuberculosis (Reproduced with permission from Rangaka et al. [22]. ©2015 Elsevier. All Rights Reserved)

level include general improvements in nutrition and housing; treatment or prevention of conditions that increase the risk of tuberculosis, such as HIV infection and diabetes; and infection control in health facilities.

The clinical epidemiology of tuberculosis involves two distinct steps: the process of becoming infected and the process of becoming ill with active disease. Risk factors for these two processes are quite different, and in approaching control of the disease it is important to be mindful of these distinctions. The principal risk factor for *M. tuberculosis* infection is exposure to someone with untreated active disease. The most easily identifiable population of those with exposure is household or other close contacts of individuals with active disease. *M. tuberculosis* is considerably less infectious than other airborne pathogens, such as chickenpox or measles, and studies of children who are household contacts of newly diagnosed adults with tuberculosis show a ~30 % prevalence of infection, and non-household contacts have a lower prevalence, in the 10–20 % range [21]. Transmission of infection outside of the home is clearly very important and contributes a large proportion of the burden of new infections in many settings, but the likelihood of such transmission is difficult to quantify. Among contacts of people with active tuberculosis, risk factors for becoming infected include the severity of the illness in the index cases, including such measures of bacillary burden as sputum smear positivity, extent of pulmonary involvement on chest x-rays, and the presence of pulmonary cavities. The environment in which exposure occurs is also important. Sharing air in closed environments with limited ventilation is more conducive to transmission.

Globally, people living in countries, regions, cities, neighborhoods, or households with a high burden of tuberculosis have the greatest risk of infection. In both high and lower burden settings, working (or studying) in an environment with a higher concentration of tuberculosis cases than in the community increases the risk of infection. Thus, health-care workers, prison staff, employees in homeless shelters, and taxi and bus drivers may be at higher risk of *M. tuberculosis* infection.

Once infection is established, risk factors for progression to disease reflect both bacillary and host susceptibility factors. Among household contacts, a greater degree of sputum smear positivity in the index case increases the likelihood of the contact progressing to active disease, suggesting that initial bacillary burden predicts risk. Despite years of study, no strain-related differences in *M. tuberculosis* have been shown to confer greater virulence. Between 5 and 8 % of individuals with recent infection progress to active disease within 2 years, though the mechanisms of their increased susceptibility is usually not apparent. Thus, recent infection is an important category of increased risk, and close contacts of tuberculosis cases should be targeted for screening and preventive therapy. Medical conditions or treatments that alter host defenses increase the risk of progressing from latent to active tuberculosis [21]. Globally, the most important of these is HIV infection, which profoundly affects host immunity and results in >100-fold risk of developing tuberculosis. Individuals with HIV infection who acquire a new *M. tuberculosis* infection have up to a 40% chance of becoming ill within 3–6 months, and people with existing latent tuberculosis who acquire HIV experience an immediate doubling of risk and ultimately develop disease at rates of 5–15% per year in the absence of antiretroviral or tuberculosis preventive therapy [22].

Other groups at increased risk of progression from latent to active tuberculosis include people with diabetes, end-stage renal disease, some cancers, and silicosis. Medical therapies that increase risk of disease include corticosteroids, tumor necrosis factor-α inhibitors, cancer chemotherapy, and immunosuppressants used for transplantation [23]. Table 1.1 lists risk factors for both acquisition of *M. tuberculosis* infection and progression to active disease. Knowledge of epidemiologic risk factors for both tuberculosis infection and progression to disease is extremely important in clinical management of individuals with signs and symptoms of active tuberculosis, as will be discussed in subsequent chapters.

TABLE 1.1 Epidemiology of tuberculosis: risk factors

For *M. tuberculosis* infection	For progression of *M. tuberculosis* infection to active disease
Close contact with an active tuberculosis case (increased risk with higher bacillary load in index case)	HIV infection
	Diabetes
	End-stage renal disease
	Silicosis
Residence in a high-burden community	Long-term corticosteroid use
Residence in congregate living facilities with a high burden of disease (prisons, long-term care facilities)	Tumor necrosis factor-a use
	Cancer chemotherapy
	Transplant medication (e.g., tacrolimus)
Working in an environment with a high burden of disease (hospitals, clinics, homeless shelters)	

References

1. Daniel TM. The history of tuberculosis. Respir Med. 2006;100:1862–70.
2. Bunyan J. The life and death of Mr. Badman. 1680. (Reprinted by Bibliolife, 2008).
3. Wilson LG. Commentary: medicine, population, and tuberculosis. Int J Epidemiol. 2005;34:521–4.
4. Vynnycky E, Fine PEM. Interpreting the decline in tuberculosis: the role of secular trends in effective contact. Int J Epidemiol. 1999;28:327–34.
5. Gagneux S. Host-pathogen coevolution in human tuberculosis. Philos Trans R Soc Lond B Biol Sci. 2012;367:850–9.
6. Schatz A, Bugie E, Waksman S. Streptomycin, a substance exhibiting antibiotic activity against Gram-positive and Gram-negative bacteria. Proc Soc Exp Biol Med. 1944;55:66–9.
7. Blumberg HM, Burman WJ, Chaisson RE, Daley CL, Etkind SC, Friedman LN, et al. American Thoracic Society/Centers for Disease Control and Prevention/Infectious Diseases Society of America: treatment of tuberculosis. Am J Respir Crit Care Med. 2003;167:603–62.
8. American Thoracic Society/Centers for Disease Control and Prevention. Targeted tuberculin testing and treatment of latent tuberculosis infection. Am J Respir Crit Care Med. 2000;161: S221–43.
9. Bloom BR, Murray CJ. Tuberculosis: commentary on a reemergent killer. Science. 1992;257(5073):1055–64.
10. Chaisson RE, Martinson NA. Perspective: Tuberculosis in Africa--combating an HIV-driven crisis. N Engl J Med. 2008;358: 1089–92.
11. Zignol M, Hosseini MS, Wright A, et al. Global incidence of multidrug-resistant tuberculosis. J Infect Dis. 2006;194(4): 479–85.
12. World Health Organization. Global tuberculosis report 2015. Geneva: World Health Organization; 2015.
13. Gandhi NR, Nunn P, Dheda K, Schaaf HS, Zignol M, van Soolingen D, Jensen P, Bayona J. Multidrug-resistant and extensively drug-resistant tuberculosis: a threat to global control of tuberculosis. Lancet. 2010;375:1830–43.

14. Karakousis PC, Bishai WR, Dorman SE. Mycobacterium tuber-culosis cell envelope lipids and the host immune response. Cell Microbiol. 2004;6(2):105–16.
15. Cole ST, Brosch R, Parkhill J, Garnier T, Churcher C, Harris D, et al. Deciphering the biology of Mycobacterium tuberculosis from the complete genome sequence. Nature. 1998;393(6685):537–44.
16. Takiff HE, Feo O. Clinical value of whole-genome sequencing of Mycobacterium tuberculosis. Lancet Infect Dis. 2015;15(9):1077–90.
17. Brites D, Gagneux S. Co-evolution of Mycobacterium tuberculo-sis and Homo sapiens. Immunol Rev. 2015;264(1):6–24.
18. Bustamante J, Boisson-Dupuis S, Abel L, Casanova JL. Mendelian susceptibility to mycobacterial disease: genetic, immunological, and clinical features of inborn errors of IFN-gamma immunity. Semin Immunol. 2014;26(6):454–70.
19. Coimbra Jr CE, Basta PC. The burden of tuberculosis in indige-nous peoples in Amazonia, Brazil. Trans R Soc Trop Med Hyg. 2007;101(7):635–6.
20. The Lubeck disaster. Science. 1930;72(1860):198–9.
21. Dowdy DW, Chaisson RE, Churchyard GJ. Tuberculosis. In: Detels R, Martin Gulliford M, Abdool Karim Q, Tan CC, editors. Oxford textbook of global public health. 6th ed. Oxford: Oxford University Press; 2015.
22. Rangaka MX, Cavalcante SC, Martinson N, Marais BJ, Thim S, Swaminathan S, Chaisson RE. Controlling the seedbeds of tuberculosis: diagnosis and treatment of tuberculosis infection. Lancet. 2015;386:2244–53.
23. Getahun H, Matteelli A, Chaisson RE, Raviglione M. Latent *Mycobacterium tuberculosis* infection. N Engl J Med. 2015;372:2127–35.

Chapter 2
Clinical Features and Diagnosis of Tuberculosis: Primary Infection and Progressive Pulmonary Tuberculosis

Petros C. Karakousis, Noton K. Dutta, and Yukari C. Manabe

2.1 Pathophysiology

More than 80 % of patients with tuberculosis (TB) manifest pulmonary findings with classical symptoms of productive cough with or without hemoptysis, fevers, night sweats, and weight loss.

The lungs represent the primary portal of entry and major target organ for *M. tuberculosis*, which is acquired by inhalation of fine evaporated mucus droplets, named droplet nuclei containing the bacilli. Small droplet nuclei containing bacilli bypass the mucociliary system and reach the alveoli [1], where they are rapidly phagocytosed by resident macro-

P.C. Karakousis (✉) • N.K. Dutta • Y.C. Manabe
Division of Infectious Diseases, Department of Medicine, Johns Hopkins University School of Medicine, Baltimore, MD, USA
e-mail: petros@jhmi.edu; ndutta1@jhmi.edu; ymanabe@jhmi.edu

J.H. Grosset, R.E. Chaisson (eds.), *Handbook of Tuberculosis*, 17
DOI 10.1007/978-3-319-26273-4_2,
© Springer International Publishing Switzerland 2017

phages. The internal pH of the macrophage phagosome drops rapidly as a result of the release of pro-inflammatory cytokines, including interferon-gamma (IFN-γ), which inhibits bacillary growth and promotes fusion with the lysosome. Additionally, IFN-γ stimulates the macrophage to release tumor necrosis factor α (TNF-α), which is important in granuloma formation and prevention of dissemination.

The T-lymphocyte response is antigen specific and is influenced by the major histocompatibility complex. This initial immune process continues for 2–12 weeks; the microorganisms continue to grow until they reach sufficient numbers to fully elicit a cell-mediated immune response, which coincides with a positive tuberculin skin test [2]. The characteristic pathological feature of the *M. tuberculosis* lesion is caseation, which derives from the Latin word for "cheese." Caseation is central to the "life cycle" of human TB infection as it may progress to liquefactive necrosis and cavitation, with the potential for drainage into the airways and transmission to patient contacts.

Typical tuberculous granulomas have a highly organized structure consisting of central necrosis surrounded by lymphocytes and fibrocytes [2]. Prominent B-cell aggregates surrounded by CD3+ T cells are found at the periphery, together with CD68+ multinucleated Langerhans cells. The recruitment of T cells, macrophages, and dendritic cells continues even without an increase in bacterial burden and during chronic infection and leads to an exaggerated immune response and tissue damage [3]. In vitro and animal data suggest that mature necrotic granulomas also contain nutrient-rich foamy macrophages, which may be a sanctuary for the bacilli [4].

Successful immune containment of infection leads to latent TB infection [5]. Latent TB infection is defined clinically by a reactive tuberculin skin test (TST), indicating a delayed-type hypersensitivity (DTH) response to intradermal injection of *M. tuberculosis*-derived purified proteins, in the absence of clinical and radiographic findings [6]. Unlike patients with

TABLE 2.1 Latent TB infection vs. active TB disease

Latent TB infection	Active TB disease
Small number of bacilli in the body (paucibacillary)	Many tubercle bacilli in the body
Tuberculin skin test reaction usually positive	Tuberculin skin test reaction usually positive
Chest X-ray usually normal	Chest X-ray usually abnormal
Sputum smears and culture negative	Sputum smears and cultures usually positive
No symptoms	Cough and constitutional symptoms, including fever, weight loss
Not infectious	Generally infectious before treatment

active pulmonary TB, latently infected individuals are not contagious (Table 2.1).

2.2   Clinical Manifestations of Primary Pulmonary Tuberculosis

Primary pulmonary TB, i.e., initial infection with *M. tuberculosis*, is classically described in infants and children under the age of 5, who have not been exposed previously to the organism. Primary TB in children is often subclinical, but may present as a unilateral pneumonia in the lower and middle lobes, often accompanied by hilar adenopathy. Pleural effusions and infiltrates are common in adolescents and young adults. Primary TB may be indistinguishable radiographically from bacterial pneumonia, especially with parenchymal lobar consolidation. Adding to the diagnostic challenge, primary TB is often paucibacillary in nature, and bacteriological confirmation is obtained by culture of sputum or bronchoalveolar lavage in only 25–30 % of cases [7]. In approximately two-thirds of cases, the parenchymal focus resolves without sequelae, although this process may take several years. Healed scars on X-ray may calcify, representing the Ghon focus.

Although primary TB is commonly viewed as a pediatric illness, it has been noted to occur in patients over the age of 50 years in many studies, perhaps due to hormonal changes in the elderly population, in whom the clinical manifestations may be protean. Thus, fever is often the only symptom, while a quarter of patients may complain of pleuritic or retrosternal pain.

2.3   Progressive Primary Tuberculosis

Failure in immune containment leads to primary progressive TB, which is seen mostly in children <5 years old or in individuals with HIV infection or other immunosuppressive conditions. Additional risk factors include nutritional status and infectious inoculum. Progressive primary TB occurs within 1–2 years after the initial infection and is often characterized by extrapulmonary involvement, with associated fevers, night sweats, and chronic weight loss.

Unlike reactivation TB, which tends to involve the apical and posterior segments of the upper lobes or the superior segment of the lower lobes, primary progressive TB tends to cause disease of the lower lobes. Pleural effusions are usually unilateral and may vary in size, occurring in approximately 40 % of adults with primary TB. Lung cavitation occurs in only 10–30 % of adults with progressive primary TB [8]. Diagnosis may be particularly difficult in cases in which there is a low bacillary load [9].

2.4   Secondary/Reactivation Tuberculosis

2.4.1   Risk Factors

Secondary TB, also known as reactivation TB or postprimary tuberculosis, usually results from reactivation of dormant tubercle bacilli many years or even decades after initial infection.

Secondary disease can occur in immunocompetent individuals despite acquisition of cellular immunity. In low-incidence countries, such as the United States, secondary TB is almost always the result of reactivation of endogenous reinfection. Reactivation of latent infection may accompany immunosuppression, such as HIV infection, uncontrolled diabetes mellitus, sepsis, renal failure, malnutrition, smoking, chemotherapy, organ transplantation, and long-term corticosteroid usage. While the lifetime risk of TB reactivation is approximately 10 % in latently infected, immunocompetent persons, for persons with HIV coinfection, the annual risk can exceed 10 % [10], and the risk of TB reactivation rises as the CD4 cell count declines [11]. Also a number of immunologic defects have been noted in patients with *M. tuberculosis* and HIV infections, including impaired T-cell proliferation, decreased cytolytic T-cell responses, deranged intracellular killing, and reduced cytokines.

Following the widespread use of TNF antagonists for the treatment of rheumatoid arthritis and other inflammatory conditions, a relationship was observed between the use of these agents and the development of granulomatous infections. Specifically, pulmonary and extrapulmonary TB was reported with significantly increased frequency among patients soon after initiation of treatment with the chimeric monoclonal antibody, infliximab [12]. Subsequently, an elevated risk of TB was found in patients treated with the TNF soluble receptor, etanercept [13], as well as other TNF antagonists (reviewed in [14]).

A characteristic feature of secondary TB is extensive necrosis with cavitation due to extensive bacillary replication, usually occurring in the apical or posterior segments of one or both upper lobes (Simon's foci), where the organisms were seeded during the primary infection [15].

2.4.2   *Clinical Signs and Symptoms of Patients with Postprimary Pulmonary Tuberculosis*

Patients with reactivation TB may have varied clinical presentations ranging from life-threatening disease to minimal complaints. In general, the disease tends to be more rapidly progressive among genetically vulnerable populations and those with acquired forms of immunosuppression. Symptoms may be predominantly respiratory in nature, including prolonged cough (≥ 2 weeks in duration), hemoptysis, and thoracic pain, and/or constitutional, such as fever, night sweats or chills, fatigue, anorexia, malaise, and weight loss.

Productive cough is almost always present with lung involvement. Damage of minor blood vessels may accompany tissue destruction, leading to the expectoration of small amounts of blood with phlegm in a third of cases with pulmonary TB. Destructive inflammation of a bronchial artery may present with massive hemoptysis in a quarter of cases and is usually associated with smear-positive and cavitary lung disease. Although uncommon (up to 5 % of cases with cavities), Rasmussen pulmonary aneurysms, which are grossly dilated pulmonary arteries adjacent to or within cavity walls, are also an important cause for massive hemoptysis in patients with TB. Finally, fistulas may develop between the bronchial and pulmonary vascular circuits, leading to hemoptysis. More important than exsanguination, massive hemoptysis poses an immediate risk for acute respiratory failure due to filling of airways and airspaces with blood. Other respiratory tract symptoms include hoarseness, which may be a sign of laryngeal disease and increased risk for transmission.

Physical examination is often unremarkable. Fever is not universally present in patients with pulmonary TB, and the percentage of patients hospitalized for TB treatment with fever ranges from 55 to 79 % [16–18]. Factors reported to be associated with fever include male sex, alcoholism, younger age, and higher burden of disease, as assessed by radiography and acid-fast staining of sputum. Since up to one-third of hospitalized patients with culture-confirmed pulmonary TB may be afebrile, the lack of fever should not exclude the diagnosis of pulmonary TB.

Adventitious breath sounds are often appreciated only with advanced lung involvement. Localized and post-tussive rales may suggest a TB-associated infiltrate, although this is an inconsistent finding. Dullness to percussion and limited thoracic excursion are often found with pleural thickening due to TB pleurisy; however, pleural friction rubs are rarely present, even when pleuritic chest pain is reported. Lymphadenopathy of the cervical and supraclavicular is rarely observed, and intrathoracic lymph nodes are usually not enlarged on chest X-ray. Similarly, hepatomegaly and splenomegaly are infrequent findings on physical examination. Clubbing of the digits is quite rare, especially among patients with new-onset pulmonary TB, but may be present in a minority of patients with chronic active TB. Cutaneous abnormalities, including erythema nodosum, erythema annulare centrifugum, and erythema induratum, are very rare.

Tuberculous empyema represents a chronic, active infection of the pleural space, usually with a large number of tubercle bacilli. Empyema is rare compared with tuberculous pleural effusions resulting from an exaggerated inflammatory response to a localized paucibacillary pleural infection with tuberculosis.

2.5   Diagnosis of Pulmonary Tuberculosis

Per the 2005 American Thoracic Society/Centers for Disease Control/Infectious Diseases Society of America guidelines [19], the diagnostic evaluation of patients for TB varies by the patient's risk and clinical characteristics (Table 2.2).

The work-up generally begins with a chest radiograph. Unlike in primary TB, where the X-ray is often unremarkable, reactivation TB often manifests with abnormalities in the upper lung zones, including fibronodular infiltrates and cavities with thick, moderately irregular walls, and lack of air-fluid levels. The earliest parenchymal finding is a heterogeneous, poorly marginated opacity situated in the apical and posterior segments of the upper lobes and the superior segments of the lower lobes, radiating outward from the hilum or in the periphery of the lung. So-called "coin" lesions are spherical and cavitary in appearance on radiograph. Early in the disease course, these findings tend to be unilateral, most commonly involving the apical/posterior segments of the right upper lobe. However, with progression of disease, chest radiography may demonstrate

TABLE 2.2 Guidelines for the evaluation of pulmonary tuberculosis in adults in five clinical scenarios

Patient and setting	Recommended evaluation
Any patient with a cough of ≥2–3 weeks' duration	Chest radiograph: If suggestive of TB, collect three sputum specimens for acid-fast bacilli (AFB) smear microscopy, culture, and nucleic acid amplification (NAA), if available
Any patient at high risk for TB with an unexplained illness, including respiratory symptoms of ≥2–3 weeks' duration	Chest radiograph: If suggestive of TB, collect three sputum specimens for AFB smear microscopy, culture, and NAA, if available
Any patient with human immunodeficiency virus (HIV) infection and unexplained cough or fever	Chest radiograph: Collect three sputum specimens for AFB smear microscopy, culture, and NAA, if available
Any patient at high risk for TB with a diagnosis of community-acquired pneumonia who has not improved after 7 days of treatment†	Chest radiograph: Collect three sputum specimens for AFB smear microscopy, culture, and NAA, if available
Any patient at high risk for TB with incidental findings on chest radiograph suggestive of TB, even if symptoms are minimal or absent	Review of previous chest radiographs, if available; collect three sputum specimens for AFB smear microscopy, culture, and NAA, if available

Source: Adapted from: ATS, CDC, IDSA. Controlling tuberculosis in the United States: recommendations from the American Thoracic Society, CDC, and the Infectious Diseases Society of America
† Patient with recent exposure to a person with a case of active TB, history of a positive test for *M. tuberculosis* infection, drug use (injection and non-injection), foreign birth and immigration from an TB endemic region in the last 5 years, residents and employees of high-risk congregate settings, membership in a medically underserved, low-income population, or a medical risk factor for TB (diabetes mellitus, prolonged corticosteroid or other immunosuppressive agent, chronic renal failure, certain hematologic malignancies, and carcinomas, weight > 10 % below ideal body weight, silicosis, gastrectomy, or jejunoileal bypass).

bilateral involvement, as well as involvement of the lower lobes following endobronchial spillage of cavity contents. The predilection of reactivation disease for the upper lobes of the lungs may be due to the higher oxygen tension of these lung zones and the obligate aerobic nature of the tubercle bacillus, although other factors likely play a greater role in this phenomenon, including the reduced pulmonary artery/capillary flow and lymph fluid generation in the upper lobes [20], the impaired intracellular killing of *M. tuberculosis* by alveolar macrophages in oxygen-rich environments relative to hypoxic environments [21], and the preferential bacillemic seeding of the upper lobes following primary infection [22].

If the radiograph is suggestive of TB, three sputum specimens for acid-fast bacilli (AFB) smear and culture are obtained. In patients with HIV or patients at high risk for TB who have failed 7 days of treatment for community-acquired pneumonia, or in patients at high risk for TB with incidental chest radiographic appearance consistent with TB, even in the absence of other symptoms, sputum specimens are taken regardless of chest radiograph appearance. An additional sputum should be obtained for rapid confirmation of *M. tuberculosis* by nucleic acid amplification testing (NAAT) in sputum smear-positive patients. NAAT allows rapid amplification of a specific target RNA or DNA sequence, which is detected using a nucleic acid probe, yielding a sensitivity and specificity of 95 and 98 %, respectively, in smear-positive patients. For sputum smear-negative patients, NAAT has a sensitivity and specificity of 75 and 88 %, respectively. Therefore, a negative NAAT is not sufficient to exclude the diagnosis of TB and should be repeated after checking for PCR inhibitors with an additional specimen.

Compared to AFB smear microscopy, NAAT assays (E-MTD or Amplicor) have the added advantage of greater positive predictive value for *M. tuberculosis* in settings where nontuberculous mycobacteria are prevalent and for rapid confirmation, with a sensitivity of 50–80 % in AFB smear-negative, culture-positive specimens, which has implications for ongoing transmission in patients suspected of having TB (Table 2.3). Xpert MTB/RIF, a newer automated NAAT platform, can identify both *M. tuberculosis* complex and rifampin resistance;

in a pooled meta-analysis of 18 studies (with TB prevalence ranging from 18.3 to 100 %), the pooled sensitivity and specificity were 89 % [95 % CI, 85–92 %] and 99 % [95 % CI, 95–99 %], respectively [23]. The Xpert MTB/RIF also addresses technical drawbacks to the previous NAAT assays; there is a decreased risk for cross contamination (self-enclosed cartridge); results are available within 2 hours, and technicians require only limited training. However, for smear-negative, culture-positive TB, the pooled sensitivity and specificity are lower, 67 % [95 % CI, 60–74 %] and 98 % [95 % CI, 97–99 %], respectively. Therefore, culture is still required for smear-negative, Xpert-negative patients.

Sputum specimens are of critical importance for the diagnosis of pulmonary TB, and every effort should be made to obtain high-quality specimens of lower respiratory tract secretions for analysis. In addition, sputum should be of adequate quantity (at least 1 ml, but preferably 3–5 ml), with proper attention to issues of infection control and proper labeling of specimens. For patients who are unable to spontaneously produce sputum, induction of cough should be attempted by inhalation of a nebulized heated saline (induced sputum). If induced sputum is not possible or is unsuccessful, an alternative is gastric aspiration, which is based on the overnight accumulation of respiratory secretions in the stomach due to

TABLE 2.3 Nucleic acid amplification tests

Test name	Sputum AFB smear positive	Sputum AFB smear negative
Enhanced amplified *Mycobacterium tuberculosis* direct test (E-MTD; GenProbe)	√ within 7 days of Rx	√ within 7 days of Rx
Amplicor *Mycobacterium tuberculosis* test (Amplicor)	√ within 7 days of Rx	N/A
Xpert MTB/RIF test (FDA approved for sputum only)	√ within 3 days of Rx	√ within 3 days of Rx

Rx treatment, *N/A* not applicable

bronchial ciliary clearance and reflexive swallowing of respiratory mucus. This technique is most effective early in the morning and should be performed prior to any beverage and food intake. If the preceding measures do not yield a diagnostic sputum specimen and the clinical suspicion for pulmonary TB or drug resistance remains high, bronchoscopy may be attempted to obtain bronchoalveolar lavage fluid, although this may have decreased sensitivity due to higher volumes. Because of the associated risks and discomfort for the patient, as well as increased risk of transmission to the health-care workers during the procedure, bronchoscopy should be reserved as a last resort for the diagnosis of pulmonary TB. Relative to bronchoscopy, sputum induction appears to be more sensitive (87 % vs. 71 %) and has a comparable negative predictive value (96 % vs. 91 %) for pulmonary TB [24].

2.6   Diagnosis of Latent Tuberculosis Infection

Currently, the diagnosis of latent TB infection is based on reactive tuberculin skin testing (TST) and/or a positive interferon-gamma release assay (IGRA) [25]. TST has lower sensitivity in diagnosing TB infection in HIV-infected individuals than in other populations. Because the sensitivity of the TST declines with progressive immunosuppression, an induration of ≥ 5 mm is considered positive in the setting of HIV infection. The TST may yield false-positive results due to vaccination with *M. bovis* BCG and/or exposure to environmental mycobacteria, but may also be falsely negative, especially in the context of HIV coinfection [26].

IGRAs detect *M. tuberculosis* exposure by measuring IFN-γ release in response to the antigens, early secreted antigenic target 6 (ESAT-6), and culture filtrate protein 10 (CFP-10), which are expressed by *M. tuberculosis* but not by *M. bovis* BCG [26, 27]. For this reason, IGRAs are thought to demonstrate superior specificity and positive predictive value for latent TB infection relative to the TST. However, other nontuberculous mycobacteria, such as *M. szulgai*, *M. kansasii*, and *M. marinum*, may cross-react with IGRAs and yield false-positive results [28]. The QuantiFERON-TB In Tube (QFT-GIT) test (Cellestis/Carnegie, Australia) has now been recommended by the CDC for the detection of *M. tuberculosis* infection [28], but was not endorsed by the WHO due to lack of data [29]. Systematic reviews have shown that another IGRA, TSPOT (Oxford Immunotec), and TST results were concordant in 77 % of HIV-infected adults but there was significant heterogeneity among individual studies [30]. The QFT-GIT alone was more effective to detect latent TB infection than TST alone and had an 81 % added value as an add-on sequential test among patients with AIDS in a city with a low TB incidence rate [31]. Long-term follow-up studies of large cohorts are required to determine if TST-negative, IGRA-positive cases represent true latent TB infection. A major limitation of the TST and IGRAs is that none of these tests is able to distinguish between latent TB infection and active disease. The ideal test would accurately identify those latently infected individuals who are at highest risk for reactivation TB for targeted preventive therapy.

2.7   Intrathoracic and Regional Spread of Tuberculosis

2.7.1   Miliary Pattern of Lung Involvement

Miliary TB results from widespread hematogenous dissemination of progressive primary infection or via reactivation of a latent focus with subsequent spread. The term "miliary" derives from the characteristic radiographic appearance of many tiny spots resembling millet seeds, which are distributed throughout the lung fields. A miliary pattern is seen in 10 % of patients with AIDS and pulmonary TB and in ~40 % of AIDS cases with extrapulmonary TB [32]. Acute miliary TB is characterized by a caseating granulomatous reaction with a smaller number of organisms than other forms of miliary disease. It is usually observed within the first 2–6 months following exposure, although progression may be more rapid in neonates and children under the age of 1 year [33]. Miliary TB may also occur in the context of reactivation, without evidence of an active primary focus. In a subset of such cases, the disease is relatively indolent and characterized by anergy and the absence of granulomas [34]. Presenting symptoms of miliary TB are nonspecific and include fever, chills, night sweats, weight loss, and anorexia. Clinical manifestations depend on the organs involved. Fulminant disease, including septic shock, acute respiratory distress syndrome, and multi-organ failure, has been described. Chest radiographs are usually normal at the onset of symptoms, and the earliest finding, seen within 1–2 weeks, may be hyperinflation of the lungs. Subsequent chest radiographs or CT scans reveal numerous 2 to 3-mm nodules in a perivascular and periseptal distribution scattered throughout the lungs. A nodular thickening of interlobular septa can result in a "beaded septum" appearance similar to that of carcinomatous lymphangitis; rarely nodules may coalesce into parenchymal consolidation or progress to acute respiratory distress syndrome. The tuberculin skin test is not useful for the diagnosis of miliary TB, as it is positive in less than 50 % of patients with this form of the disease due to tuberculin anergy. The sputum smear is positive in approximately 30 % of patients with miliary TB, but can be positive in 70 % of cases with lung cavitation [35]. Blood cultures may be positive in a small percentage of miliary TB cases, particularly in the setting of HIV coinfection. Diagnosis is based on biopsy and culture of affected sites. Diagnostic delays due to negative tests and nonspecific signs and symptoms contribute to the high mortality, which can exceed 25 % in adults.

2.7.2   Tuberculous Pleurisy

Tuberculous pleurisy is among the most common forms of thoracic TB, accounting for about 4 % of TB cases in the United States and 20 % of those in South Africa. Patients with pleural TB tend to be younger than patients with pulmonary TB. Immune status contributes to the pathogenesis of tuberculous pleurisy, as the incidence is higher in HIV-infected individuals than in those who are uninfected. Primary TB pleurisy is thought to result from rupture of a subpleural caseous focus into the pleural space, leading to pleural infection and a local delayed-type hypersensitivity response to mycobacterial antigens. The most common presenting symptoms are pleuritic chest pain and nonproductive cough. Additional symptoms may include fever, night sweats, weight loss, malaise, and dyspnea, which may vary in severity based on the size of the effusion. Chest radiography usually reveals a small-to-moderate unilateral pleural effusion. Acid-fast smears and cultures of pleural fluid are positive in only 30 % of cases, and the diagnostic yield can be improved by pleural biopsy. Depending on the cutoff value used, adenosine deaminase activity (ADA) in the pleural fluid may have diagnostic utility with a high positive predictive value. A meta-analysis of Xpert MTB/RIF testing of pleural fluid for *M. tuberculosis* detection reveals that it performs relatively poorly compared to standard culture with a sensitivity of 46.4 % (95 % CI, 26.3–67.8 %) and specificity of 99.1 % (95 % CI, 95.2–99.8 %) [36].

2.7.3   Regional Tuberculosis Lymphadenitis

Depending on the geographical region surveyed, almost half of non-pulmonary TB cases are characterized by regional lymphadenitis. Cervical lymph nodes may become involved by direct extension from the buccal mucosa or upper airways. Based on radiological and clinical characteristics, TB lymphadenitis may be divided into three categories: nodular, diffuse, and sclerosing. TB lymphadenitis usually presents as a painless, slowly progressive swelling of a single group of nodes, and in 85 % of cases involvement is unilateral [37]. The cervical lymph nodes are most commonly affected, whereas axillary lymph node involvement is relatively rare. In young children, airway compromise secondary to enlarging and eroding peribronchial or paratracheal lymph nodes may lead to paroxysmal cough, wheezing, and dyspnea. However, in adults, mediastinal lymphadenitis is usually asymptomatic. Uncommon presentations include progressive jaundice due to biliary obstruction, dysphagia due to cervical adenitis, and chyluria due to obstruction of the thoracic duct. In addition to swollen lymph nodes, the typical TB-associated constitutional signs and symptoms may be present, which may confuse the clinical picture with malignancy. Physical examination may reveal discrete, rubbery, nontender lymphadenopathy. TST is positive in 90 % of cases of TB lymphadenitis, while chest radiographs are abnormal in 30 % cases. Tuberculous lymphadenitis is routinely diagnosed by lymph node biopsy for histology, acid-fast stain, and mycobacterial cultures. In cases lacking acid-fast organisms, it may be challenging to distinguish among the various etiologies of granulomatous lymphadenitis. PCR of lymph node tissue for *M. tuberculosis* may improve the diagnostic yield in patients with a clinical suspicion of tuberculous lymphadenitis [38]. Off-label use of Xpert MTB/RIF on lymph node aspirates revealed a pooled sensitivity of 83.1 % (95 % CI, 71.4–90.7 %) and specificity of 93.6 % (95 % CI, 87.9–96.8 %) compared to culture [36].

References

1. Riley RL, Wells WF, Mills CC, Nyka W, McLean RL. Air hygiene in tuberculosis: quantitative studies of infectivity and control in a pilot ward. Am Rev Tuberc. 1957;75:420–31.
2. Dannenberg Jr AM. Roles of cytotoxic delayed-type hypersensitivity and macrophage-activating cell-mediated immunity in the pathogenesis of tuberculosis. Immunobiology. 1994;191:461–73.
3. Tsai MC, Chakravarty S, Zhu G, Xu J, Tanaka K, Koch C, Tufariello J, Flynn J, Chan J. Characterization of the tuberculous granuloma in murine and human lungs: cellular composition and relative tissue oxygen tension. Cell Microbiol. 2006;8:218–32.
4. Peyron P, Vaubourgeix J, Poquet Y, Levillain F, Botanch C, Bardou F, Daffe M, Emile JF, Marchou B, Cardona PJ, de Chastellier C, Altare F. 2008. Foamy macrophages from tuberculous patients' granulomas constitute a nutrient-rich reservoir for M. tuberculosis persistence. PLoS Pathog 4:e1000204.
5. Dutta NK, Karakousis PC. Latent tuberculosis infection: myths, models, and molecular mechanisms. Microbiol Mol Biol Rev. 2014;78:343–71.

6. Horsburgh Jr CR, Rubin EJ. Clinical practice. Latent tuberculosis infection in the United States. N Engl J Med. 2011;364: 1441–8.

7. Sia IG, Wieland ML. Current concepts in the management of tuberculosis. Mayo Clin Proc. 2011;86:348–61.

8. Woodring JH, Vandiviere HM, Fried AM, Dillon ML, Williams TD, Melvin IG. Update: the radiographic features of pulmonary tuberculosis. AJR Am J Roentgenol. 1986;146:497–506.

9. Mathew P, Kuo YH, Vazirani B, Eng RH, Weinstein MP. Are three sputum acid-fast bacillus smears necessary for discontinuing tuberculosis isolation? J Clin Microbiol. 2002;40:3482–4.

10. Selwyn PA, Hartel D, Lewis VA, Schoenbaum EE, Vermund SH, Klein RS, Walker AT, Friedland GH. A prospective study of the risk of tuberculosis among intravenous drug users with human immunodeficiency virus infection. N Engl J Med. 1989;320: 545–50.

11. Markowitz N, Hansen NI, Hopewell PC, Glassroth J, Kvale PA, Mangura BT, Wilcosky TC, Wallace JM, Rosen MJ, Reichman LB. Incidence of tuberculosis in the United States among HIV-infected persons. The Pulmonary Complications of HIV Infection Study Group. Ann Intern Med. 1997;126:123–32.

12. Keane J, Gershon S, Wise RP, Mirabile-Levens E, Kasznica J, Schwieterman WD, Siegel JN, Braun MM. Tuberculosis associated with infliximab, a tumor necrosis factor alpha-neutralizing agent. N Engl J Med. 2001;345:1098–104.

13. Mohan AK, Cote TR, Block JA, Manadan AM, Siegel JN, Braun MM. Tuberculosis following the use of etanercept, a tumor necrosis factor inhibitor. Clin Infect Dis. 2004;39:295–9.

14. Cantini F, Niccoli L, Goletti D. Tuberculosis risk in patients treated with non-anti-tumor necrosis factor-alpha (TNF-alpha) targeted biologics and recently licensed TNF-alpha inhibitors: data from clinical trials and national registries. J Rheumatol Suppl. 2014;91:56–64.

15. Hunter RL. Pathology of post primary tuberculosis of the lung: an illustrated critical review. Tuberculosis (Edinb). 2011;91:497–509.

16. Barnes PF, Chan LS, Wong SF. The course of fever during treatment of pulmonary tuberculosis. Tubercle. 1987;68:255–60.

17. Kiblawi SS, Jay SJ, Stonehill RB, Norton J. Fever response of patients on therapy for pulmonary tuberculosis. Am Rev Respir Dis. 1981;123:20–4.

18. Iseman MD. A clinician's guide to tuberculosis. Philadelphia: Lippincott Williams and Wilkins; 2000.

19. Anonymous. American Thoracic Society/Centers for Disease Control and Prevention/Infectious Diseases Society of America: controlling tuberculosis in the United States. Am J Respir Crit Care Med. 2005;172:1169–227.
20. Dock W. Apical localization of phthisis; its significance in treatment by prolonged rest in bed. Am Rev Tuberc. 1946;53:297–305.
21. Meylan PR, Richman DD, Kornbluth RS. Reduced intracellular growth of mycobacteria in human macrophages cultivated at physiologic oxygen pressure. Am Rev Respir Dis. 1992;145:947–53.
22. Balasubramanian V, Wiegeshaus EH, Taylor BT, Smith DW. Pathogenesis of tuberculosis: pathway to apical localization. Tuber Lung Dis. 1994;75:168–78.
23. Steingart KR, Schiller I, Horne DJ, Pai M, Boehme CC, Dendukuri N. Xpert(R) MTB/RIF assay for pulmonary tuberculosis and rifampicin resistance in adults. The Cochrane database of systematic reviews. 2014;1:Cd009593.
24. Anderson C, Inhaber N, Menzies D. Comparison of sputum induction with fiber-optic bronchoscopy in the diagnosis of tuberculosis. Am J Respir Crit Care Med. 1995;152:1570–4.
25. Salgame P, Geadas C, Collins L, Jones-Lopez E, Ellner JJ. Latent tuberculosis infection – revisiting and revising concepts. Tuberculosis (Edinb). 2015;95:373–84.
26. Pai M, Denkinger CM, Kik SV, Rangaka MX, Zwerling A, Oxlade O, Metcalfe JZ, Cattamanchi A, Dowdy DW, Dheda K, Banaei N. Gamma interferon release assays for detection of Mycobacterium tuberculosis infection. Clin Microbiol Rev. 2014; 27:3–20.
27. Schluger NW. Advances in the diagnosis of latent tuberculosis infection. Semin Respir Crit Care Med. 2013;34:60–6.
28. Mazurek GH, Jereb J, Vernon A, LoBue P, Goldberg S, Castro K. Updated guidelines for using Interferon Gamma Release Assays to detect Mycobacterium tuberculosis infection – United States, 2010. MMWR Recomm Rep. 2010;59:1–25.
29. Anonymous. Use of tuberculosis interferon-gamma release assays (IGRAs) in low- and middle-income countries: policy statement. Geneva; 2011.
30. Cattamanchi A, Smith R, Steingart KR, Metcalfe JZ, Date A, Coleman C, Marston BJ, Huang L, Hopewell PC, Pai M. Interferon-gamma release assays for the diagnosis of latent tuberculosis infection in HIV-infected individuals: a systematic review and meta-analysis. J Acquir Immune Defic Syndr. 2011;56: 230–8.

31. Souza JM, Evangelista Mdo S, Trajman A. Added value of QuantiFERON TB-gold in-tube for detecting latent tuberculosis infection among persons living with HIV/AIDS. Biomed Res Int. 2014;2014:294963.
32. Shafer RW, Kim DS, Weiss JP, Quale JM. Extrapulmonary tuberculosis in patients with human immunodeficiency virus infection. Medicine (Baltimore). 1991;70:384–97.
33. Perry TL. Natural history and pathogenesis of miliary and meningeal tuberculosis in children; analysis of 163 cases. Pediatrics. 1950;5:988–97.
34. Slavin RE, Walsh TJ, Pollack AD. Late generalized tuberculosis: a clinical pathologic analysis and comparison of 100 cases in the preantibiotic and antibiotic eras. Medicine (Baltimore). 1980;59:352–66.
35. Maartens G, Willcox PA, Benatar SR. Miliary tuberculosis: rapid diagnosis, hematologic abnormalities, and outcome in 109 treated adults. Am J Med. 1990;89:291–6.
36. Denkinger CM, Schumacher SG, Boehme CC, Dendukuri N, Pai M, Steingart KR. Xpert MTB/RIF assay for the diagnosis of extrapulmonary tuberculosis: a systematic review and meta-analysis. Eur Respir J. 2014;44:435–46.
37. Mert A, Tabak F, Ozaras R, Tahan V, Ozturk R, Aktuglu Y. Tuberculous lymphadenopathy in adults: a review of 35 cases. Acta Chir Belg. 2002;102:118–21.
38. Mirza S, Restrepo BI, McCormick JB, Fisher-Hoch SP. Diagnosis of tuberculosis lymphadenitis using a polymerase chain reaction on peripheral blood mononuclear cells. Am J Trop Med Hyg. 2003;69:461–5.

Chapter 3
Treatment of Pulmonary Tuberculosis

Susan Dorman and Amita Gupta

3.1 Treatment of Active Tuberculosis Disease

3.1.1 Principles

Antibiotic treatment of active tuberculosis disease has three main goals. The first is to rapidly reduce the population of replicating bacteria in order to resolve symptoms/signs, prevent death, and prevent transmission of infection. The second is to eliminate the subpopulations of persisting bacteria that could cause relapse after stopping treatment and thereby to achieve durable cure. The third is to prevent the emergence of drug resistance during therapy.

Combination therapy – the simultaneous use of multiple antibiotics – is required to achieve these goals. Moreover, the

_____

S. Dorman (✉)
Department of Medicine, Johns Hopkins University School of Medicine, 1550 Orleans St, Rm 1M-12, Baltimore, MD 21231, USA
e-mail: DSUSAN1@JHMI.EDU

A. Gupta
Center for Clinical Global Health Education, Johns Hopkins University, 600 North Wolfe Street, Phipps 540B, Baltimore, MD 21287, USA
e-mail: agupta25@jhmi.edu

J.H. Grosset, R.E. Chaisson (eds.), *Handbook of Tuberculosis*,
DOI 10.1007/978-3-319-26273-4_3,
© Springer International Publishing Switzerland 2017

individual drugs that comprise the combination matter and are not necessarily interchangeable. For drug-susceptible tuberculosis, the composition and duration of the recommended regimen are supported by decades of clinical trials and practice (reviewed in [1, 2]). Rifampin and pyrazinamide (PZA) form the backbone of current 6-month duration "short-course" chemotherapy. Rifampin and some other rifamycins have potent, unique sterilizing activity through their action against subpopulations of slowly metabolizing bacilli that are thought to be responsible for relapse after treatment cessation. PZA, a prodrug converted by host and bacterial enzymes to the active form, pyrazinoic acid, also has sterilizing activity. The 6-month duration of "short-course" tuberculosis treatment depends on the sterilizing activities of the rifamycins and PZA – if these drugs are absent from a regimen for whatever reason (e.g., resistance, intolerance), then cure requires longer treatment. Isoniazid acts to rapidly reduce the burden of replicating bacteria early in the treatment course; later on during continuation phase, it helps to prevent emergence of resistance to rifampin. Ethambutol has modest antituberculosis activity, and its main role in the current first-line regimen is to protect against acquisition of additional drug resistance in the event that a patient's *M. tuberculosis* already has (clinically unrecognized) resistance.

The decision to initiate treatment is a critical one. Microbiological confirmation always should be sought in order to firmly establish a species-level diagnosis as well as drug susceptibility profile. In the absence of or while awaiting microbiological confirmation, the decision to initiate treatment should take into account multiple factors including the level of clinical suspicion based on other medical and epidemiological information, likelihood of death or significant morbidity from tuberculosis if present, potential toxicities of treatment, and public health factors. It is worth reemphasizing that a diagnosis of active tuberculosis is *not* excluded by negative smears for acid-fast bacilli and/or negative results on a tuberculin skin test or interferon gamma release assay.

3.1.2   Classes of Available Antituberculosis Drugs

Antituberculosis drugs are grouped into five groups based on evidence of efficacy, potency, experience of use, and drug class (Table 3.1) [3, 4]. "First-line" Group 1 drugs are those recommended for use in the treatment of drug-susceptible tuberculosis. "Second-line" drugs (Groups 2, 3, 4) are generally reserved for drug-resistant tuberculosis. Third-line drugs (Group 5) have unclear efficacy and/or unclear role in tuberculosis treatment, although for certain Group 5 drugs, this may more reflect a shortcoming in our knowledge than shortcomings of the drugs themselves. The antituberculosis drugs most commonly encountered in US practice as well as bedaquiline, a novel agent recently approved by the US FDA for certain tuberculosis indications, are described below.

Isoniazid

Isoniazid inhibits *M. tuberculosis* mycolic acid synthesis through its action on the enoyl-[acyl-carrier-protein] reductase. Isoniazid acts on actively replicating bacilli – this is manifest as robust early bactericidal activity (decline in bacillary colony-forming units during the initial few days of therapy), and as a result, isoniazid has an important role early on in treatment. Resistance to isoniazid appears to develop via two main pathways, namely, mutations in the *katG* gene and in the promoter region of the *inhA* gene.

Rifamycins

Rifamycins inhibit bacterial transcription through inhibition of the beta subunit of the bacterial RNA polymerase. Rifamycins have activity against poorly replicating "persister" *M. tuberculosis* bacilli, manifest as sterilizing activity that eradicates bacilli and cures that patient. The rifamycins appear to be unique in this regard, and there is no other single drug that can replace the rifamycin in short-course chemotherapy for drug-

TABLE 3.1 Classification of antituberculosis drugs

First-line drugs	**Group 1**
	Rifamycins
	   Rifampin, rifampicin
	   Rifapentine
	   Rifabutin
	Isoniazid
	Pyrazinamide
	Ethambutol

Second-line drugs	**Group 2**
	Injectable aminoglycosides
	   Streptomycin
	   Amikacin
	   Kanamycin
	Injectable polypeptides
	   Capreomycin
	   Viomycin

	Group 3 (Fluoroquinolones) Moxifloxacin Levofloxacin Gatifloxacin Ofloxacin Ciprofloxacin
	Group 4 Cycloserine Para-aminosalicylic acid Terizidone Ethionamide Prothionamide
Third-line drugs	**Group 5** Clofazimine Linezolid Amoxicillin plus clavulanate Imipenem plus cilastatin Clarithromycin Thioacetazone

susceptible tuberculosis. Therefore clinically the implications of "loss" of rifamycins from a patient's regimen (due to resistance or intolerance) are grave. Rifampin (rifampicin) is the most commonly used rifamycin. Rifapentine is a cyclopentyl ring-substituted rifamycin that, compared with rifampin, has a longer half-life and generally lower minimum inhibitory concentration against *M. tuberculosis*. Rifampin and rifapentine have similar side effect profiles; both are potent inducers of hepatic metabolic enzymes and have similar drug-drug interactions vis-à-vis spectrum and intensity. Rifabutin is not as potent an inducer of cytochrome P450 enzymes and can be used in some circumstances (e.g., with some antiretroviral drugs) in which neither rifampin nor rifapentine can be used reliably. Challenges with using rifabutin include narrow therapeutic window and the need to dose adjust rifabutin when used with certain other drugs (this adds complexity and can increase the risk of rifamycin resistance). Resistance to the rifamycins is conferred almost solely by mutations in the *rpoB* gene.

Pyrazinamide

Pyrazinamide is an important albeit puzzling drug. It is a pro-drug that needs to be activated by the mycobacterial enzyme nicotinamidase, named pyrazinamidase (PZase) to its active form, pyrazinoic acid (POA). After its activation, it is generally accepted that POA is expelled from the mycobacterial cell by an efflux pump and is protonated in the extracellular environment. Upon reentry into the bacterial cell, this proton is released, decreasing the cytoplasmic pH and thus causing lethal damage through several possible mechanisms, including membrane disruption, inhibition of fatty acid synthetase, and inhibition of trans-translation of *Mycobacterium tuberculosis*. Mutations in the bacterial pncA gene that encodes the pyrazinamidase appear responsible for most pyrazinamide resistance. Mutations in the rpsA gene have less frequently been implicated in pyrazinamide resistance. During the treatment of pulmonary tuberculosis, the activity of pyrazinamide is greatest, or at least most consequential, when administered during the first 2 months of treatment; continuation of pyrazinamide after intensive phase appears to confer no demonstrable clinical benefit, and omission of pyrazinamide from a pulmonary tuberculosis treatment regimen reduces the regimen's potency such that 9 months or more of treatment are required for durable cure. Thus pyrazinamide, the rifamycins, and isoniazid are the key drugs in short-course treatment of drug-susceptible pulmonary tuberculosis.

Ethambutol

Ethambutol inhibits mycobacterial arabinogalactan biosynthesis and has bacteriostatic activity against *M. tuberculosis*. In patients being initiated on first-line tuberculosis therapy, ethambutol is recommended unless the patient's isolate is already known to be fully susceptible to isoniazid, rifampin, and pyrazinamide. Ethambutol's main role in first-line tuberculosis treatment is to prevent emergence of resistance to the rifamycin and PZA in the event that unrecognized resistance to isoniazid is already present. Ethambutol can rarely cause optic neuritis, manifest by decreased visual acuity and/or diminished red/green color discrimination; high daily doses, prolonged use, and renal insufficiency are risk factors. Unlike other antituberculosis drugs, ethambutol is cleared mainly by the kidneys, and the dosing interval should be increased to three times per week (not daily) in adults with creatinine clearance <30 ml/min and those receiving conventional intermittent hemodialysis (administer three times per week after hemodialysis).

Fluoroquinolones

Fluoroquinolones inhibit bacterial DNA gyrase and DNA topoisomerase. Moxifloxacin and levofloxacin are substantially more potent against *M. tuberculosis* than ciprofloxacin, which should not be used. Moxifloxacin and levofloxacin are preferred over ofloxacin. Fluoroquinolone resistance is not uncommon, and therefore the susceptibility of a patient's *M. tuberculosis* isolate to fluoroquinolones should be confirmed if a drug from this class is to be used. Resistance to fluoroquinolones is most commonly conferred by mutations in the *gyrA* gene; *gyrB* mutations can also have clinical significance.

Aminoglycosides

Aminoglycosides, which inhibit protein synthesis, have been used for parenteral treatment of tuberculosis since streptomycin was developed in the mid-twentieth century. There is abundant clinical trial evidence from the mid-twentieth century to support streptomycin for tuberculosis treatment. However, oral ethambutol has replaced parenteral streptomycin in first-line therapy for drug-susceptible tuberculosis because of ethambutol's ease of administration and tolerability. Furthermore streptomycin resistance is now not uncommon. If an aminoglycoside is indicated, the choice of agent generally depends on availability, *M. tuberculosis* resistance profile, and antibiotic side effect profile. Amikacin has excellent activity against *M. tuberculosis*, and measurement of serum amikacin concentrations is generally readily feasible in the USA, although clinical experience suggests that administration of intramuscular amikacin is more painful than is administration of intramuscular streptomycin. The molecular basis of *M. tuberculosis* resistance to aminoglycosides (and the cyclic peptide capreomycin) is complex and incompletely understood, and there are several different patterns of cross-resistance. All of the aminoglycosides, as well as capreomycin, are toxic to the eighth cranial nerve and therefore can cause both auditory and vestibular toxicity. Effects are usually cumulative and may be irreversible (especially vestibular toxicity). In general, streptomycin has more vestibular toxicity and less auditory toxicity than amikacin or kanamycin. Patients treated with aminoglycosides should have monthly audiograms and assessments for vestibular toxicity.

Bedaquiline

Bedaquiline is a diarylquinoline that inhibits the *c* subunit of the *M. tuberculosis* ATP synthase, thereby decreasing bacterial intracellular ATP levels. Bedaquiline has activity against dormant and actively replicating bacteria. Bedaquiline (Sirturo, Janssen Therapeutics) was approved by the US FDA in 2012 for the treatment of pulmonary MDR-TB in adults (in combination with other antituberculosis drugs) when an effective treatment regimen cannot otherwise be provided. Bedaquiline has black box warnings about the QT prolongation that can occur with its use, as well as the increased risk of death observed in the bedaquiline group compared with the placebo group in a clinical trial. In the USA, bedaquiline is available by prescription only from healthcare providers associated with qualified tuberculosis care centers – information can be obtained from public health departments, by phone at 1-855-691-0963 or at https://www.sirturo.com.

3.1.3   Recommended Regimens

For tuberculosis disease presumed to be susceptible to isoniazid, rifampin, PZA, and ethambutol, the preferred initial regimen is comprised of two months ("intensive phase") of isoniazid, rifampin, PZA, and ethambutol [5]. Ethambutol can be omitted from the intensive phase in the (uncommon) event that the patient's isolate has already been confirmed microbiologically to be fully susceptible to isoniazid, rifampin, and PZA. To minimize the risk of isoniazid-associated peripheral neuropathy, pyridoxine (vitamin B6) supplementation should be given with each dose of isoniazid to patients with other conditions associated with neuropathy (e.g., diabetes, HIV infection, renal failure, alcoholism, nutritional deficiencies, certain chemotherapies) as well as to pregnant women and breastfeeding women.

The "continuation phase" follows intensive phase. The standard continuation phase is comprised of isoniazid plus rifampin, with pyridoxine administered as described above [5]. Continuation phase typically is administered for 4 months (18 weeks), resulting in an overall treatment duration of 6 months (18 weeks). However, as described below the duration of continuation phase should be increased in certain situations.

Recommended adult drug dosages are shown in Table 3.2. With regard to dosing frequency, the antimicrobial activity

TABLE 3.2 Antituberculosis drugs and doses for DAILY treatment

	How supplied	Adult dose for DAILY treatment (CrCl>30 ml/min)	Pediatric dose for DAILY treatment	Common adverse reactions and other information
Conventional First-line antituberculosis drugs				
Isoniazid	Tablet 50 mg, 100 mg, 300 mg Elixir 50 mg/5 ml Aqueous solution 100 mg/ml for intravenous or intramuscular injection	5 mg/kg (typically 300 mg)	10–15 mg/kg	*Adverse Reactions:* Relatively common: GI upset, asymptomatic elevation of transaminases, peripheral neurotoxicity (use pyridoxine) Uncommon but potentially severe: hepatitis, allergic/ hypersensitivity reactions, CNS toxicity (seizures, encephalopathy, psychosis, optic neuritis) Isoniazid is a weak monoamine oxidase inhibitor and can induce tyramine reactions. Signs/symptoms (typical onset 2–3 h after eating tyramine-rich foods) can include flushing, hypertension, headache, blurred vision, nausea/vomiting, chest pain, stroke symptoms *Adult dosing if CrCl <30 ml/min or intermittent hemodialysis:* No change *Clinically significant common DDIs (see text):* Phenytoin, carbamazepine, diazepam, triazolam *Other comments:* Coadministration of glucose or lactose decreases isoniazid absorption therefore (a) use low-glucose food such as sugar-free pudding if tablets to be crushed and (b) elixir contains sorbitol, causes diarrhea

TABLE 3.2 (continued)

	How supplied	Adult dose for DAILY treatment (CrCl>30 ml/min)	Pediatric dose for DAILY treatment	Common adverse reactions and other information
Rifampin	Capsule 150 mg, 300 mg Aqueous solution for intravenous injection	10 mg/kg (typically 600 mg)	10–20 mg/kg	*Adverse Reactions:* Relatively common: harmless red discoloration of secretions, GI upset, asymptomatic elevation of transaminases Uncommon but potentially severe: hepatitis (typically with cholestatic indices), allergic/hypersensitivity reactions (including flu-like symptoms, interstitial nephritis, thrombocytopenia, hemolytic anemia) *Adult dosing if CrCl <30 ml/min or intermittent hemodialysis:* No change *Clinically significant common DDIs:* Multiple, see Table 3.5 *Other comment:* Powder from capsules may be suspended for oral administration.

PZA	Tablet 500 mg, scored	25 mg/kg (maximum 2000 mg daily) Using whole tabs: Weight 40–55 kg 1000 mg PZA Weight 56–75 kg 1500 mg PZA Weight 76–90 kg 2000 mg PZA	35 mg/ kg (range 30 mg/kg to 40 mg/kg) (maximum 2000 mg daily)	*Adverse Reactions:* Relatively common: skin rash, asymptomatic elevations in serum uric acid, arthralgias, GI upset, asymptomatic elevation of transaminases Uncommon but potentially severe: hepatitis, allergic/ hypersensitivity reactions *Adult dosing if CrCl <30 ml/min or intermittent hemodialysis:* 25–35 mg/kg/dose given three times per week (not daily) Administer after HD *Other comments:* Maximum daily dose 2000 mg, regardless of body weight
Ethambutol	Tablet 100 mg, 400 mg	20 mg/kg (maximum 1600 mg daily) Using whole tabs: Weight 40–55 kg 800 mg EMB Weight 56–75 kg 1200 mg EMB Weight 76–90 kg 1600 mg EMB	20 mg/kg (range 15 mg/kg to 25 mg/kg) (maximum 1600 mg)	*Adverse Reactions:* Relatively common: none; low rates of rash, GI upset; not hepatotoxic Uncommon but potentially severe: retinal toxicity (usually first perceived as decrease in color perception) *Adult dosing if CrCl <30 ml/min or intermittent hemodialysis:* 15–25 mg/kg/dose given three times per week (not daily) Administer after HD *Other comments:* Maximum daily dose 1600 mg, regardless of body weight

(continued)

TABLE 3.2 (continued)

	How supplied	Adult dose for DAILY treatment (CrCl>30 ml/min)	Pediatric dose for DAILY treatment	Common adverse reactions and other information
Vitamin B6 (pyridoxine)	Tablet	25 or 50 mg		*Adverse Reactions:* Relatively common: none (low rates of GI upset, headache) Uncommon but potentially severe: sensory neuropathy *Other comments:* Administer when an INH-containing regimen is used Administer pyridoxine to breastfeeding infant if mother is receiving INH
Other commonly used antituberculosis drugs				
Rifabutin	Capsule 150 mg	5 mg/kg (typically 300 mg)	Appropriate dose not established but estimated at 5 mg/kg	*Adverse Reactions:* Relatively common: harmless red discoloration of secretions, loss of taste, *C. difficile* colitis Uncommon but potentially severe: neutropenia, thrombocytopenia, uveitis *Adult dosing if CrCl <30 ml/min:* dose reduction of 50 % recommended *Adult dosing for intermittent hemodialysis:* not known with certainty; 300 mg may be appropriate *Clinically significant common DDIs:* Multiple, see Table 3.5

| Rifapentine | Tablet 150 mg, film-coated | | *Adverse Reactions:* Relatively common: harmless red discoloration of secretions, GI upset, asymptomatic elevation of transaminases Uncommon but potentially severe: hepatitis (typically with cholestatic indices), allergic/hypersensitivity reactions (including flu-like symptoms, interstitial nephritis, thrombocytopenia, hemolytic anemia) *Adult dosing if CrCl <30 ml/min or intermittent hemodialysis:* no change *Clinically significant common DDIs:* Multiple, see Table 3.5 |
| Moxifloxacin | Tablet 400 mg Aqueous solution 400 mg/ 250 ml for intravenous injection | 400 mg | *Adverse Reactions:* Relatively common: GI upset, taste disturbance Uncommon but potentially severe: tendinopathy, ventricular arrhythmia, hepatitis, allergic/hypersensitivity reactions *Adult dosing if CrCl <30 ml/min or intermittent hemodialysis:* no change *Clinically significant common DDIs:* Absorption of moxifloxacin is markedly decreased by divalent cations (calcium, iron, zinc), sucralfate, chewable form of didanosine. If these must be used, then separate administration of these drugs from moxifloxacin administration by at least 2 h. Many antacids, nutritional supplements, vitamin/mineral supplements contain divalent cations |

Optimal dose not known.

(continued)

TABLE 3.2 (continued)

	How supplied	Adult dose for DAILY treatment (CrCl > 30 ml/min)	Pediatric dose for DAILY treatment	Common adverse reactions and other information
Levofloxacin	Tablet 250 mg, 500 mg, 750 mg Aqueous solution (500 mg vials) for intravenous injection	500–1000 mg	Optimal dose not established, but clinical data support 15–20 mg/kg (Schaaf 2015)	*Adverse Reactions:* Relatively common: GI upset, dizziness, headache, insomnia Uncommon but potentially severe: tendinopathy, ventricular arrhythmia, hepatitis, allergic hypersensitivity reactions, hypoglycemia *Adult dosing if CrCl <30 ml/min or intermittent hemodialysis:* 750–1000 mg/dose given three times per week (not daily) Administer after HD *Clinically significant common DDIs:* As above for moxifloxacin

Note: Intermittent hemodialysis assumes hemodialysis three times weekly. For peritoneal dialysis, data to guide dosing and frequency are limited; experts recommend starting with doses recommended for intermittent hemodialysis and verify adequacy of dosing by measuring serum concentrations. Data are limited for daily hemodialysis (e.g., daily short home hemodialysis) and continuous hemodialysis – consultation with an expert is advised

CrCl creatinine clearance, *DDI* drug-drug interactions

and therefore presumably the efficacy of first-line tuberculosis drugs is greater when administered every day than when administered less frequently. If daily directly observed therapy (DOT) is difficult to achieve, then three-times-weekly DOT is preferred over twice-weekly DOT. Twice-weekly and once-weekly regimens should not be used in HIV-positive patients or patients with cavitary disease (Table 3.3).

3.1.4   Duration of Treatment

The following recommended durations of treatment apply to individuals with drug-susceptible pulmonary tuberculosis who are treated with and adherent with an intensive phase comprised of isoniazid, rifampin (or rifabutin), and PZA and continuation phase comprised of isoniazid and rifampin (or rifabutin):

I. Pulmonary tuberculosis: The standard total duration of treatment is 6 months. In order to reduce the risk of relapse, the treatment duration should be 9 months (i.e., continuation phase should be extended to 7 months) in individuals who have cavitation on initial or follow-up chest radiograph *plus* sputum culture positive for *M. tuberculosis* from sputum obtained at the time of completion of the intensive phase of treatment [6, 7].

II. Lymph node tuberculosis: a regimen of 6-month duration is recommended.

III. Pleural tuberculosis: a regimen of 6-month duration is recommended. Randomized clinical trials do not support the routine use of adjunctive systemic corticosteroids for pleural tuberculosis [8–11]. Tuberculous empyema, which is rare, can occur when a pulmonary cavity ruptures into the pleural space and requires drainage in addition to antituberculosis chemotherapy; the optimum duration of treatment has not been well established.

TABLE 3.3 Drug regimens for culture-positive pulmonary tuberculosis caused by drug-susceptible organisms

Regimen	Intensive phase Drugs	Intensive phase Interval and doses[a] (minimum duration)	Continuation phase Drugs	Continuation phase Interval and doses[a,b] (minimum duration)	Range of total doses	Comments	Relative potency
1	INH RIF PZA EMB	Seven days per week for 56 doses (8 weeks), or 5 days per week for 40 doses (8 weeks)	INH RIF	Seven days per week for 126 doses (18 weeks), or 5 days per week for 90 doses (18 weeks)	182–130	This is the preferred regimen for patients with newly diagnosed pulmonary tuberculosis	Greater
2	INH RIF PZA EMB	Seven days per week for 56 doses (8 weeks), or five days per week for 40 doses (8 weeks)	INH RIF	Three times weekly for 54 doses (18 weeks)	110–94	Preferred alternative regimen in situations in which more frequent DOT during continuation phase is difficult to achieve	
3	INH RIF PZA EMB	Three times weekly for 24 doses (8 weeks)	INH RIF	Three times weekly for 54 doses (18 weeks)	78	Use with caution in patients with HIV and/or cavitary disease	
4	INH RIF PZA EMB	Seven days per week for 14 doses then twice weekly for 12 doses, or 5 days per week for 15 doses then twice weekly for 12 doses	INH RIF	Twice weekly for 36 doses (18 weeks)	63–62	Do not use twice weekly therapy in HIV-positive patients or patients with cavitary disease	Lesser

INH isoniazid, *RIF* rifampin, *PZA* pyrazinamide, *EMB* ethambutol

[a]When DOT is used, drugs may be given 5 days per week and the necessary number of doses adjusted accordingly. Although there are no studies that compare five with seven daily doses, extensive experience indicates this would be an effective practice. DOT should be used when drugs are administered for fewer than 7 days per week

[b]Patients with cavitation on initial chest radiograph and positive cultures at completion of 2 months of therapy should receive a 7-month (31 week) continuation phase

IV. Pericardial tuberculosis: a regimen of 6-month duration is recommended. While it has been longstanding clinical practice to administer adjunctive systemic corticosteroids, a recent large randomized placebo-controlled clinical trial did not find a difference in the combined endpoint of mortality, constrictive pericarditis, or cardiac tamponade [12]. However, subgroup analyses suggested a benefit of corticosteroids in preventing constrictive pericarditis. Therefore, the routine use of adjunctive corticosteroids in the treatment of pericardial tuberculosis is not recommended. Use of corticosteroids in patients at high risk for inflammatory complications (e.g., those with early signs of constriction, or large pericardial effusions, or high levels of inflammatory cells or markers in pericardial fluid) may be appropriate.

V. Abdominal tuberculosis: a regimen of 6-month duration is recommended.

VI. Genitourinary tuberculosis: a regimen of 6-month duration is recommended.

VII. Tuberculosis of the bone, joint, and/or spine: 6–9 months of treatment is recommended; the authors generally treat for 9 months. Uncomplicated cases of spinal tuberculosis usually can be treated without surgical intervention; surgery should be considered in patients with ongoing infection or clinical deterioration despite treatment, neurological deficits, cord compression, or spine instability.

VIII. Tuberculous meningitis: the optimum duration of therapy has not been well established; most experts treat for 9–12 months. Adjunctive corticosteroid therapy (e.g., dexamethasone given over a 6–8 week period) confers a mortality benefit and is recommended [13, 14].

IX. Disseminated tuberculosis: for tuberculosis involving multiple sites and for miliary tuberculosis a standard 6-month regimen is typically sufficient provided that the central nervous system is not involved.

3.1.5   Practical Aspects

Directly Observed Therapy

Directly observed therapy (DOT) refers to the practice of observing the patient swallow tuberculosis medications. DOT is one of a number of practices (see below) that can help to maximize the likelihood of successful and safe completion of tuberculosis treatment. DOT can help to ensure medication adherence and should be used when tuberculosis treatment is administered intermittently rather than daily. Importantly, DOT can also enable early identification of medication toxicities or worsening of tuberculosis, as well as linkage to other social/health services from which the patient may benefit. In the USA, DOT is normative practice for tuberculosis treatment and is usually coordinated through the local health department.

Case Management and Role of the Health Department

Tuberculosis disease is a reportable condition, and all patients diagnosed with tuberculosis should be reported to the local health department. For tuberculosis, an infectious disease that is transmitted through the respiratory route and that has public health implications, the responsibility for successful completion of treatment lies with the healthcare provider rather than or at least as much as with the patient. Health departments have legal authority to control tuberculosis and therefore also have responsibility for assuring access by patients to appropriate tuberculosis care. Health departments can differ in their capacity to provide direct clinical care, and therefore the responsibilities of various healthcare providers should be defined clearly. Most health departments provide case management – the coordination of care on the behalf of an individual being treated for tuberculosis – that includes assessment of and reduction of potential barriers to treatment adherence, assessment of psychosocial and other needs and linkage to services, provision of information about tuberculosis to the patient (and others, if relevant), and monitoring of tuberculosis clinical response and potential toxicities. Local health departments typically perform public health activities including contact investigations (to identify other individuals with *M. tuberculosis* infection or disease).

Monitoring for Efficacy and Toxicity During Treatment

General guidelines for monitoring are provided in Table 3.4. Additional assessments may be clinically indicated based on individual patient comorbidities and concomitant medications and if tuberculosis involves extrapulmonary sites.

Common Adverse Drug Reactions

Adverse drug reactions are relatively common even when first-line antituberculosis drugs are used. Patients should be counseled about common and serious drug reactions and where/how they can get medical attention should they experience reactions. DOT and case management practices may provide convenient mechanisms for ongoing education about drug reactions, as well as early recognition and close management of any reactions that occur.

Table 3.5 provides information about common adverse drug reactions as well as about reactions that are less common but can be serious and should be recognized promptly. Importantly, for most patients, most of the relatively mild side effects will lessen or resolve after several weeks of treatment, without stopping antituberculosis drugs. The patient's perspective on which drug is causing or associated with their side effect(s) can be enlightening. As in treatment of other medical conditions, eliminating or minimizing side effects is critical; additional facets relevant in tuberculosis treatment are associated with the limited armamentarium of potent antituberculosis drugs, and the communicable nature of the disease such that stopping treatment due to side effects can impact public health as well as the patient's health.

Table 3.4 Assessments recommended before treatment initiation and while on treatment for pulmonary tuberculosis patients treated with first-line drugs

	Baseline	Month 1	Month 2	Month 3	Month 4	Month 5	Month 6[a]	Month 7[a]	Month 8[a]	End of treatment
Symptom review for clinical response, toxicity[b]	✓	✓	✓	✓	✓	✓	✓	✓	✓	✓
Adherence review		✓	✓	✓	✓	✓	✓	✓	✓	✓
Review of concomitant medicines	✓	✓	✓	✓	✓	✓	✓	✓	✓	✓[g]
Weight	✓	✓	✓	✓	✓	✓	✓	✓	✓	✓
Vision assessment	✓	✓	If ethambutol continued, then perform monthly while on ethambutol							
Liver chemistries	✓	Obtain monthly or periodically if abnormal at baseline, in patients who use alcohol or are on other potentially hepatotoxic medications, have history of liver disease, or are HIV positive. Obtain if signs and/or symptoms of hepatotoxicity during tuberculosis treatment								
Creatinine	✓	Obtain periodically if abnormal at baseline or as clinically indicated due to comorbidities								
Platelet count	✓									
HIV test	✓									
Hepatitis B & C screen[c]	✓									
Diabetes screen	✓									

Chest X-ray or other chest imaging	√	√[f]	√[d]	√[e]
Sputum smear and culture	√[f]	√[f]	√[f]	Obtain monthly while on treatment, until two consecutive monthly cultures are negative. In practice this usually means that monthly cultures are done at least through month 4
Rapid molecular test on sputum	√			
Drug susceptibility testing	√			Repeat DST if a specimen that was obtained after completing 3 months of treatment is culture positive for *M. tuberculosis*

[a]For patients in whom therapy is extended to 9 months total duration

[b]Cough, fatigue, fever, sweats, appetite; nausea, vomiting, abdominal discomfort, jaundice, dark urine, rash, arthralgias, peripheral neuropathy; others as indicated clinically

[c]Hepatitis B and C screens should be performed in patients with risk factors (e.g., injection drug use, HIV infection, birth in Asia or Africa)

[d]If baseline cultures are negative, then obtain chest X-ray or other chest imaging at completion of 2 months of treatment as component of assessment of treatment response. Optional in other patients

[e]Optional although most programs perform an end-of-treatment chest X-ray as it can be very useful in establishing a new "baseline" for an individual

[f]Three sputum specimens typically are obtained around baseline. Two sputum specimens typically are obtained at completion of intensive phase in order to guide duration of continuation phase (4 vs. 7 months). Additional sputum specimens may be helpful during intensive phase to assess for treatment response

[g]At the end of treatment, special attention should be paid to the potential need for adjusting doses of any concomitant medications (e.g., warfarin) for which the dose was adjusted previously to compensate for drug-drug interactions with antituberculosis drugs; additional monitoring (e.g., prothrombin time, international normalized ratio in the case of warfarin) may be required since enzyme inductive/inhibitory typically resolve gradually over about 2 weeks

Drug-Drug Interactions

There are a number of clinically relevant, commonly encountered drug-drug interactions involving the rifamycins, isoniazid, and fluoroquinolones (Table 3.6). Importantly, Table 3.6 and the paragraphs below address only concomitant medications that are very commonly used; omission from the table or discussion below does *not* imply that a concomitant medication has no clinically significant interaction with antituberculosis medications. For all patients, all medications and supplements should be reviewed for drug-drug interactions prior to initiating antituberculosis drugs and then periodically thereafter (Table 3.6).

I. *Rifamycins*. Rifamycins induce several drug metabolism pathways including the cytochrome P450 system. Therefore rifamycins reduce the serum concentrations of many other drugs, potentially decreasing the therapeutic activity of the other drug(s). Rifampin and rifapentine are more potent enzyme inducers than rifabutin. Rifamycin enzyme induction takes about 2 weeks to reach steady state, and thus the effects of a rifamycin on another drug may not be apparent immediately; careful dose adjustment of the other drug(s) and clinical and/or laboratory monitoring may be required during the first several weeks of therapy. Similarly, rifamycin inductive effects resolve over about 2 weeks once the rifamycin is stopped, and thus careful dose adjustment (of the other drugs) and monitoring may also be required during that transition. For a patient with rifampin-susceptible tuberculosis, the use of a rifamycin is always desirable from a tuberculosis disease perspective due to this drug class' critical and seemingly unique sterilizing ability, which allows short-course therapy. However, in clinical situations in which the consequences of rifamycin drug-drug interactions are potentially severe, expert consultation should be obtained in order to assist with risk-benefit assessments and identification of alternate treatment approaches for tuberculosis or the relevant comorbidity. Examples of such clinical situations include organ transplant recipients, indi-

TABLE 3.5 Adverse reactions that can be due to first-line and commonly used antituberculosis drugs

Adverse drug reaction	Commonly implicated drugs	Management considerations
Red-tinged secretions	Rifamycins	Additional clinical assessments that may be indicated: none. Clinically harmless, resolves when drug stopped; may permanently stain contact lenses. Patient education usually sufficient.
Diarrhea	Elixir form of isoniazid Fluoroquinolones	Additional clinical assessments that may be indicated: consider testing for *Clostridium difficile* colitis; consider lactose intolerance if recent diet change.
		If due to isoniazid elixir (formulated with sorbitol) then consider change to isoniazid tablets (can be crushed in low-glucose/low-lactose food).
		Most antituberculosis drugs can rarely cause (noninfectious) antibiotic-associated diarrhea, although ethambutol is a very unlikely cause. Conservative management usually sufficient – maintain hydration; consider antimotility agents if *C. difficile* colitis excluded; lactobacillus or yogurt may be helpful.
		Antimotility agents (adult doses): loperamide (Imodium) 2–4 mg po initially then 1–2 mg after each loose stool, to max dose of 8–16 mg/day. Loperamide can be used intermittently. Loperamide should not be used daily.

(continued)

Table 3.5 (continued)

Adverse drug reaction	Commonly implicated drugs	Management considerations
GI upset	Isoniazid, rifamycins, PZA, fluoroquinolones	Additional clinical assessments that may be indicated: Liver chemistries (ALT, AST, bilirubin, alk phos); physical exam; history (relationship to timing of administration of TB drugs, other hepatotoxins). Consider pregnancy in females with nausea/vomiting GI upset *not* associated with hepatotoxicity is common, especially early in TB treatment, and usually amenable to one or more of following strategies: light snack before TB drugs administered, antacids (do not administer divalent cations with fluoroquinolones), change to daily therapy if receiving intermittent therapy, administration at bedtime. Antiemetics that may be useful if conservative measures do not work: Ondansetron (Zofran) 8 mg po given 30 min prior to TB drugs (8 mg po can also be given 8 h after the dose of TB drugs if symptoms persist); metoclopramide (Reglan) 10–20 mg po every 4–6 h as needed; promethazine (Phenergan) 12.5–25 mg po given 30 min prior to TB drugs and every 6 h as needed. GI upset associated with elevated transaminases and/or hepatitis: see below.

Elevated liver transaminases and/or hepatitis		Additional clinical assessments that may be indicated: testing for viral hepatitis (Hepatitis A, B, and C in all patients; EBV, CMV, and HSV in immunosuppressed patients); patient interview to determine if patient is drinking alcohol or using other hepatotoxic drugs (e.g. acetominophen and/or acetominophen-containing products, lipid-lowering agents, some herbal supplements). Most clinicians stop hepatotoxic tuberculosis drugs when the ALT level is 3 times or greater the upper limit of normal in the presence of hepatitis symptoms, or 5 times or greater the upper limit of normal in the absence of hepatitis symptoms. Additional information is available at http://www.thoracic.org/statements/resources/mtpi/hepatotoxicity-of-antituberculosis-therapy.pdf
Skin flushing, or pruritis without rash	Rifamycins PZA Isoniazid (can cause tyramine reaction)	Additional clinical assessments that may be indicated: History as to timing of symptom onset related to TB drug ingestion and to specific food intake. Rifamycin and PZA reactions usually occur 2–3 h after dosing, and usually involve face/scalp. Tyramine reaction typically occurs 2–3 h after eating tyramine-rich foods (See Table Table 3.2) Due to rifamycins or PZA: usually resolves over time. If severe or bothersome, consider antihistamines given before administration of TB drugs: diphenhydramine (Benadryl and generics) 25–50 mg po; hydroxyzine (Atarax) 25 mg po; loratadine (Claritin) 10 mg po Tyramine reaction: educate patient to avoid tyramine-rich foods including aged cheeses, cured meats, sauerkraut, kimchi, soy sauce, fava beans.

(continued)

TABLE 3.5 (continued)

Adverse drug reaction	Commonly implicated drugs	Management considerations
Mild rash, usually with pruritis	Any Isoniazid can cause acneiform flares.	Additional clinical assessments that may be indicated: History to assess for other potential etiologies including other new drugs, scabies, contact dermatitis. Perform physical exam to assess for mucous membrane involvement, petechiae, lymphadenopathy, wheezing, and fever. Consider obtaining liver chemistries and basic metabolic profile, complete blood cell count with differential Mild rash and pruritis are relatively common especially early in treatment, may resolve spontaneously after several weeks (without stopping TB drugs), and usually can be managed conservatively while continuing TB drugs. The following may be helpful for mild rash and pruritis: diphenhydramine (Benadryl and generics) 25–50 mg po prior to administration of TB drugs and then every 4–6 h as needed; hydroxyzine (Atarax) 25 mg po prior to administration of TB drugs; loratadine (Claritin) 10 mg po prior to administration of TB drugs.

Hives and urticaria without anaphylaxis, DRESS, or Stevens-Johnson syndrome	Any	Additional clinical assessments that may be indicated: Evaluate for life-threatening hypersensitivity reactions including liver chemistries and basic metabolic profile, complete blood cell count with differential; perform physical exam to assess for mucous membrane involvement, petechiae, lymphadenopathy, wheezing, fever Hives and urticaria can be caused by any of the TB drugs. *All potentially responsible agents should be stopped immediately.* Antihistamines (as above) with or without oral corticosteroids (prednisone 10–20 mg po daily) may be helpful. If the patient is severely ill due to TB and interim TB treatment is considered necessary, then an expert should be consulted Once the reaction resolves, drug rechallenge can be considered in order to facilitate treatment with the most potent regimen that is safe and tolerated. If there is reason to suspect that a certain drug caused the initial reaction, then that drug should not be used. Otherwise, the most important drug typically is started first, and other drugs are added one at a time every 3 or 4 days.

(continued)

TABLE 3.5 (continued)

Adverse drug reaction	Commonly implicated drugs	Management considerations
Life-threatening hypersensitivity reactions: Anaphylaxis; Drug Reaction with Eosinophilia and Systemic Symptoms (DRESS); Stevens-Johnson syndrome	Any	Additional clinical assessments that may be indicated: Stop all TB drugs immediately. Hospitalization typically indicated. Obtain expert consultation for management of hypersensitivity reaction and for TB management.

| Joint discomfort | PZA (arthralgias) Fluoroquinolones (tendinopathy) | Additional clinical assessments that may be indicated: serum uric acid measurement. Mild arthralgias are relatively commonly associated with PZA. Conservative management (salicylates or nonsteroidal anti-inflammatories) usually sufficient. Avoid acetaminophen due to potential for hepatotoxicity. PZA-induced acute gout is rare. If clinical picture consistent with acute gout, then hold PZA, treat gout. Individual risk-benefit assessment as to whether to resume PZA after controlling gout flare Fluoroquinolone-associated tendinopathy is rare. Achilles tendon is most commonly affected. Risk factors include advanced age, corticosteroid use, renal insufficiency, possibly duration of fluoroquinolone use. Tendinopathy characterized by pain, swelling, inflammation at site. Signs of tendon rupture may include an audible "pop" at time of rupture, bruising, immobility of joint. Ultrasound or MRI to evaluate. Stop fluoroquinolone. |
| Peripheral neuropathy | Isoniazid | Add pyridoxine 50 mg daily if not already being administered with isoniazid. Weigh risks vs. benefits of continuing isoniazid. |

(continued)

TABLE 3.5 (continued)

Adverse drug reaction	Commonly implicated drugs	Management considerations
Irritability, seizure, psychosis	Isoniazid Fluoroquinolones	Isoniazid-associated CNS toxicity is substantially less common than peripheral nerve toxicity. If isoniazid is the likely cause, then stop isoniazid; supplemental pyridoxine prudent CNS effects from fluoroquinolones are relatively common but usually mild (e.g., irritability, insomnia, nightmares, dizziness). Management depends on severity of CNS effects, availability of other TB therapeutic options. Levofloxacin tends to have fewer CNS effects than moxifloxacin.
Visual acuity change or change in color vision	Ethambutol	Additional clinical assessments that may be indicated: ophthalmological evaluation. Discontinue ethambutol.

TABLE 3.6 Drugs in common use that can have clinically significant drug-drug interactions with antituberculosis drugs

Concomitant medication and/or drug class	Interacting antituberculosis drug	Management considerations
HIV-1 protease inhibitors: lopinavir/ritonavir, darunavir/ritonavir, atazanavir, atazanavir/ritonavir	Rifamycins	Double dose lopinavir/ritonavir can be used with rifampin but toxicity is increased. Do not use rifampin with other protease inhibitors. Rifabutin preferred with protease inhibitors; for ritonavir-boosted protease inhibitors use rifabutin 150 mg once daily.
HIV non-nucleoside reverse transcriptase inhibitors: nevirapine, efavirenz, rilpivirine, etravirine	Rifamycins	Rifampin decreases the serum concentrations of all NNRTIs. Rilpivirine and etravirine should not be given with rifampin. If nevirapine is used with rifampin, then the lead-in nevirapine dose of 200 mg daily should be omitted and nevirapine administered at 400 mg daily. If efavirenz is used with rifampin, many experts recommend an efavirenz dose of 600 mg daily, although the US FDA recommends increasing the efavirenz dose to 800 mg daily in patients >60 kg. Rifabutin should not be given with rilpivirine. Rifabutin can be used with etravirine and nevirapine at the usual doses. If efavirenz is used with rifabutin then the rifabutin dose should be increased to 600 mg daily, and thus rifampin is preferred.

(continued)

Table 3.6 (continued)

Concomitant medication and/or drug class	Interacting antituberculosis drug	Management considerations
HIV Integrase strand transfer inhibitors: raltegravir, dolutegravir, elvitegravir	Rifamycins	Rifabutin can be used with raltegravir, dolutegravir, elvitegravir. Do not use rifampin with elvitegravir. If raltegravir used with rifampin, then increase the dose of raltegravir to 800 mg twice daily. If dolutegravir used with rifampin, then increase the dose of dolutegravir to 50 mg every 12 h.
HIV CCR5 inhibitors: maraviroc	Rifamycins	Rifampin should not be used with maraviroc. Rifabutin can be used with maraviroc.
Warfarin	Rifamycins	Monitor prothrombin time and/or INR; increased warfarin dose may be required. When the rifamycin is stopped, en sure close monitoring of anticoagulation (INR); warfarin dose reduction almost always required after the rifamycin is stopped.
Estrogens, progesterones	Rifamycins	A nonhormonal contraception method should be used to prevent pregnancy.
Levothyroxine	Rifamycins	Monitor TSH. Increased levothyroxine dose may be required.
Methadone	Rifamycins	RIF and RPT can precipitate methadone withdrawal; methadone dose may need to be increased.

Azole antifungals	Rifamycins	RIF and RPT significantly decrease voriconazole levels – concomitant use is contraindicated.
Caspofungin	Rifamycins	RIF and RPT decrease caspofungin plasma concentrations; monitor clinically; caspofungin dose increase may be required.
Corticosteroids	Rifamycins	Monitor clinically; corticosteroid dose increase may be required.
Cyclosporine, tacrolimus, sirolimus	Rifamycins	RIF and RPT generally not recommended; rifabutin can be used with close monitoring of immunosuppressant levels.
Calcium channel blockers (including but not necessarily limited to: verapamil, nifedipine, diltiazem, felodipine, nisoldipine, amlodipine)	Rifamycins	Clinical monitoring recommended; may require calcium channel blocker dose increase or alternative cardiovascular agent.
Beta blockers (e.g., atenolol, labetalol, propranolol, metoprolol, nadolol)	Rifamycins	Clinical monitoring recommended; may require beta blocker dose increase or alternative cardiovascular agent.
Losartan	Rifamycins	Clinical monitoring recommended; may require losartan dose increase or alternative cardiovascular agent.

(continued)

TABLE 3.6 (continued)

Concomitant medication and/or drug class	Interacting antituberculosis drug	Management considerations
Digoxin, digitoxin	Rifamycins	Clinical and therapeutic drug monitoring recommended. May require increased digoxin dose.
Phenytoin	Rifamycins	Clinical and therapeutic drug monitoring recommended. May require increased phenytoin dose.
Lamotrigine	Rifamycins	Clinical and therapeutic drug monitoring recommended. May require increased lamotrigine dose.
Statin hypolipidemics (including but not necessarily limited to simvastatin, fluvastatin, atorvastatin, lovastatin, pravastatin)	Rifamycins	Clinical monitoring recommended. May require alternative hypolipidemic agent.
Sulfonylurea hypoglycemic (e.g., tolbutamide, chlorpropamide, glyburide, glimepiride, repaglinide)	Rifamycins	Monitor blood glucose. May require sulfonylurea dose increase or alternative hypoglycemic agent.
Haloperidol, quetiapine, clozapine	Rifamycins	Clinical monitoring recommended; may require psychotropic dose increase or alternative psychotropic agent.

Benzodiazepines (e.g., diazepam, triazolam)	Rifamycins	Clinical monitoring recommended; may require psychotropic dose increase or alternative psychotropic agent.
Buspirone, bupropion	Rifamycins	Clinical monitoring recommended; may require psychotropic dose increase or alternative psychotropic agent.
Phenytoin	Rifamycins, isoniazid	Isoniazid can increase serum levels of phenytoin and rifampin can decrease serum levels of phenytoin; clinical monitoring recommended.
Carbamazepine	Isoniazid	Isoniazid can increase the concentration of carbamazepine to the point of toxicity – clinical and therapeutic drug monitoring recommended; may require carbamazepine dose increase.
Benzodiazepines metabolized by oxidation (e.g., diazepam, triazolam)	Rifamycins, isoniazid	Isoniazid can increase serum levels of these benzodiazepines and rifampin can decrease serum levels; clinical monitoring recommended.
Benzodiazepines metabolized by conjugation (e.g., oxazepam)	Rifamycins	Clinical monitoring recommended; may require psychotropic dose increase or alternative psychotropic agent.

(continued)

TABLE 3.6 (continued)

Concomitant medication and/or drug class	Interacting antituberculosis drug	Management considerations
Theophylline	Rifamycins	Clinical and therapeutic drug monitoring recommended. May require increased theophylline dose. (Note: ciprofloxacin increases theophylline concentrations).
Calcium, iron, zinc (e.g., in nutritional supplements, antacids)	Moxifloxacin, levofloxacin	Consider stopping divalent cation. If concomitant use required then separate administration of divalent cation and fluoroquinolone by at least 2 h.
Sucralfate	Moxifloxacin, levofloxacin	Consider stopping sucralfate or changing to another agent. If concomitant use required then separate administration of divalent cation and fluoroquinolone by at least 2 h.
Didanosine chewable/buffered tablets or pediatric suspension	Moxifloxacin, levofloxacin	Consider alternative agents or other didanosine formulation (didanosine enteric bead "EC" formulation can be concomitantly administered with fluoroquinolones).

Note: Absence of a concomitant medication from this list DOES NOT imply that there is no clinically significant drug-drug interaction with antituberculosis drugs. Each of a patient's concomitant medications should be checked against each of the antituberculosis drugs planned for administration viduals with HIV, individuals anticoagulated with warfarin, and individuals receiving azole antifungals for serious infection. Rifabutin can be used in place of rifampin or rifapentine in some instances, notably with some HIV protease inhibitors and with cyclosporine. When initiating a rifamycin, it is prudent to always check a patient's concomitant medications for drug-drug interactions.

II. *Isoniazid*. Isoniazid inhibits a number of cytochrome P450 isoenzymes. Therefore isoniazid can increase the serum concentrations of some drugs including carbamazepine, phenytoin, and benzodiazepines metabolized by oxidation (e.g., diazepam and triazolam); clinical and/or laboratory monitoring is prudent. When isoniazid is administered with a rifamycin during combination therapy, the enzyme induction effects of the rifamycin tend to outweigh the enzyme inhibition effects of isoniazid, such that the net effect tends to be reduced in serum concentrations of drugs such as carbamazepine and phenytoin. Isoniazid is a weak inhibitor of monoamine oxidase and rarely can precipitate tyramine reactions.

Therapeutic Drug Monitoring

Therapeutic drug monitoring (TDM) includes the measurement of drug concentrations in blood as a means of assessing whether a given dosing approach may be "appropriate." The role of TDM in tuberculosis management has not been well defined. At present there is insufficient evidence to support routine TDM in all tuberculosis patients under treatment. However, there is emerging consensus among experts that TDM may be helpful in informing the need for dose adjustment in certain situations [15]. These include patients at risk for malabsorption of antituberculosis drugs (e.g., gastroparesis, short bowel syndrome, chronic diarrhea with malabsorption, extensive GI surgery), patients at risk for drug-drug interactions that could compromise antituberculosis drug activity, diabetes mellitus, renal insufficiency such that dose adjustments have been made to accommodate renal function, peritoneal dialysis, daily home hemodialysis, critically ill patients on continuous renal replacement, patients with poor response to tuberculosis treatment despite demonstrated drug susceptibility, and patients on second-line tuberculosis drugs. For most tuberculosis drugs, the relationships between drug exposure and efficacy on the one hand and drug exposure and toxicity on the other hand are poorly defined, such that drug concentrations must be interpreted with caution.

Treatment Failure

Treatment failure is defined as persistently positive or newly positive cultures (for *M. tuberculosis*) after 4 months of treatment in a patient on treatment. For patients with treatment failure, a recent *M. tuberculosis* isolate should be sent for DST to first- and second-line drugs, additional sputum specimens should be obtained for testing including smear and culture, and chest imaging should be performed. Potential reasons for treatment failure should be addressed, including nonadherence (e.g., missed DOT doses, spitting out pills, nonadherence in the setting of self-supervised treatment), unrecognized drug resistance, malabsorption (e.g., due to GI surgery, diabetes, antacids/other interacting substances). If the patient is doing well clinically, then the possibility of laboratory cross contamination or a specimen labeling error should also be explored. Appropriate public health measures should be taken if the patient is assessed to be infectious.

Of note, clinical assessment of response to therapy should be performed regularly during the entire course of treatment, not just at completion of 4 months. Patients who are responding poorly or slowly should be evaluated to determine the cause, ideally before they reach the point of treatment failure. In appropriately treated patients, response times and trajectory will vary depending on a number of factors (e.g., extent of pulmonary disease), but in general most patients have clear subjective improvement and at least slight weight gain by about one month into treatment; about three-quarters of patients convert sputum cultures (liquid media) to negative by completion of 2 months of treatment, and almost all convert sputum cultures to negative by completion of 3 months of treatment.

A single drug should never be added to a failing regimen, since resistance to the newly added drug can occur. A clinician experienced in the management of drug-resistant tuberculosis should be consulted. If drug resistance is suspected, the patient is seriously ill, or the sputum smear is positive, then empiric treatment with a regimen likely to be active (e.g., containing at least three new drugs against which resistance is thought to be unlikely) should be started and continued until results of susceptibility tests are available to guide treatment.

Recurrence

Recurrence refers to the scenario in which a patient who had become and remained culture-negative while on treatment subsequently becomes culture positive (or has clinical and/or radiographic deterioration) after completion of therapy. Recurrence can be caused by the same *M. tuberculosis* strain as originally identified ("relapse") or can be the result of exogenous reinfection with a different strain. Risk factors for relapse include extensive cavitary tuberculosis, positive sputum cultures at the time of completion of 2 months of treatment, nonadherence with treatment, malabsorption, suboptimal treatment regimen, and being underweight [6, 7]. Exogenous reinfection appears to be most common in immunosuppressed individuals in hyperendemic settings [16]. In patients with suspected recurrence, multiple additional specimens should be obtained for smear and culture including DST; rapid molecular DST may help to guide initial treatment decisions. Chest imaging should be performed. If tuberculosis has not yet been microbiologically confirmed, then other clinically relevant evaluations should also be performed to evaluate for tuberculosis and to exclude other etiologies for the presenting signs/symptoms.

A clinician experienced in the management of drug-resistant tuberculosis should be consulted. Management should be individualized and will depend on the level of suspicion for tuberculosis recurrence, the patient's clinical condition, available microbiologic and epidemiologic information, prior tuberculosis treatment history, and in some instances public health implications.

Drug Resistance

Drug resistance can be transmitted ("primary") or acquired ("secondary"). Transmitted resistance occurs when an individual is infected with *M. tuberculosis* bacilli that already are resistant. Acquired resistance can occur and amplify in an individual when that individual's tuberculosis treatment is inadequate (e.g., drugs are not absorbed, incorrect drugs are selected, substandard drugs are used, and nonadherence with therapy), and the risk is heightened when the bacillary burden is large such as occurs in cavitary pulmonary tuberculosis. Any large drug-susceptible population of *M. tuberculosis* contains bacilli with drug-resistant mutations that appear spontaneously at an average frequency of about 1 per 10^6 bacilli. To prevent selection of resistant bacilli and the amplification of drug resistance, the basis of tuberculosis chemotherapy is the combination of several active drugs. As long as multiple microbiologically active drugs are appropriately administered, the selection of drug-resistant mutants does not occur, and clinically significant drug resistance does not develop. Multidrug-resistant tuberculosis (MDR-TB) is caused by *M. tuberculosis* bacilli that are resistant to at least isoniazid and rifampin. Extensively drug-resistant tuberculosis is a subset of MDR-TB in which the bacilli also are resistant to any fluoroquinolone plus at least one of three injectable second-line drugs (i.e., amikacin, kanamycin, or capreomycin). Patients with suspected or confirmed drug-resistant tuberculosis should be managed in consultation with a clinician with experience in the treatment of drug-resistant tuberculosis. Molecular drug susceptibility testing should be used in combination with conventional culture-based phenotypic drug susceptibility testing to guide regimen selection.

3.2   Treatment of Latent Tuberculosis Infection

3.2.1   Principles

Latent tuberculosis infection (LTBI) is defined as a state of persistent bacterial viability, immune control, and no evidence of clinical manifestations of active TB disease. It is estimated that one-third of the world's population is infected with *M. tuberculosis* and therefore at some risk of developing TB disease and transmitting *M. tuberculosis* to others. The aim of LTBI treatment is to prevent an individual's progression to active TB disease, toward goals of reducing individual morbidity and on a population level reducing the reservoir of latently infected persons. As with any medical intervention, the potential benefits of treatment need to be weighed against the potential risks. The risk of an individual's progression from latent to active TB is determined by host, environmental, and bacterial factors. However, neither the tuberculin skin test nor interferon gamma release assays can reliably classify an individual's risk for progression from latent to active TB. Therefore, programmatic approaches to LTBI treatment generally take into account the underlying local/regional epidemiology of TB as well as resource availability and cost-effectiveness. Hence, LTBI treatment guidelines can differ from setting to setting, and readers are encouraged to consult their setting-specific guidelines documents. This review provides general principals and information, as well as current (at the time of writing) recommendations from the US CDC and the WHO.

Risk Groups

Two types of risk can be considered. The first is an individual's risk of progressing to active TB disease if already infected with *M. tuberculosis*. The second is an individual's risk of having been infected with *M. tuberculosis*; since the risk of progression to active disease is greatest during the first 2 years after infection, special emphasis is placed on identification of individuals with recent (i.e., within approximately 2 years) *M. tuberculosis* infection.

Risk factors for progression to active TB disease (if already infected) include:

- Close contact with a person with active pulmonary TB
- Age less than approximately 5 years old
- Positive test for LTBI (TST or IGRA)
- Recent conversion of TST or IGRA from negative to positive (i.e., recent *M. tuberculosis* infection)
- HIV infection
- Treatment with tumor necrosis factor-alpha inhibitors
- Treatment with glucocorticoids
- Receipt of hematologic or organ transplant
- Renal failure
- Silicosis
- Diabetes
- Smoking
- Malnutrition
- Fibrotic changes consistent with prior TB on chest radiograph

Risk factors for having been infected recently with *M. tuberculosis* can vary considerably from setting to setting. The following risk factors are relevant to much of the USA:

- Contact with a person with active pulmonary TB
- Recent immigration from a country that has a high TB burden
- Healthcare workers
- Prisoners and correctional facility staff
- Homeless adults
- Illicit drug users

Whom to Treat

The general framework is that the decision of whom to test and treat for LTBI is based on identifying who would benefit from treatment of LTBI. Except in rare circumstances, the decision to test for LTBI is a decision to treat if the LTBI test is positive. The presence of active TB disease should be excluded before LTBI treatment is initiated, for the health benefit of the patient and in order to avoid amplification of *M. tuberculosis* resistance. Recommendations from the US CDC, which are directed toward US-based practitioners, are provided in Table 3.7 [17, 18]. Guidance from the WHO is also summarized below.

I. WHO LTBI treatment guidance for high and upper middle-income countries with a TB incidence <100 per 100,000 population per year [19]

It is strongly recommended to test and treat LTBI in people living with HIV, adult and child contacts of pulmonary TB cases, patients initiating antitumor necrosis factor treatment, patients receiving dialysis, patients preparing for organ or hematological transplantation, and patients with silicosis. Other populations that may benefit from testing and treating LTBI but for whom the WHO recommendation is conditional (according to TB epidemiology and resource availability) include prisoners, homeless persons, illicit drug users, healthcare workers, and immigrants from high TB burden countries.

II. WHO LTBI treatment guidance for resource-limited countries and other middle-income countries with higher TB incidence (i.e., > 100 per 100,000 population per year)

Persons living with HIV and children below 5 years of age who are household contacts or close contacts of people with TB and who, after an appropriate clinical evaluation are found not to have active TB but have LTBI should be treated for LTBI [20]. In addition, in resource-limited settings in which there is high TB incidence and transmission, HIV-positive adults and HIV-positive adolescents who have an unknown or positive TST (or/and IGRA) and in whom active TB disease has been ruled out, should receive LTBI treatment (for at least 36 months) [21]. For other risk groups described above, there is little guidance from WHO, but many practitioners do test and treat for LTBI on a case-by-case basis.

Table 3.7 Groups who should be given high priority for LTBI treatment[a]

Treat regardless of TST/IGRA test results	Treat if the IGRA is positive or/and the TST induration is ≥ 5 mm	Treat if the IGRA is positive or/and the TST induration is ≥ 10 mm
HIV-positive persons who in addition have been recent close contacts of an individual with active pulmonary TB disease	HIV-positive persons Recent contacts of a TB case Persons with fibrotic changes consistent with prior TB on chest radiograph Organ transplant recipients Recipients of TNF-alpha inhibitor therapy Patients receiving immunosuppressant therapy equivalent to 15 mg/day of prednisone for one month or more	Recent (within the past 5 years) immigrants from high TB prevalence countries Injection drug users Mycobacteriology laboratory workers Children younger than 4 years of age Children and adolescents exposed to adults at high risk for TB Residents & employees of high-risk congregate settings (e.g., correctional facilities, nursing homes, hospitals/healthcare facilities, homeless shelters) Persons with clinical conditions that put them at risk of progression to active TB if infected (diabetes; chronic renal failure; silicosis; leukemia/lymphoma; carcinoma of the head, neck, or lung; weight loss of >10 % of ideal body weight; prior gastrectomy or jejunoileal bypass)

[a]Persons with no known risk factors for TB may be considered for treatment of LTBI if they have a positive IGRA result or/and TST induration ≥ 15 mm. However, targeted TB testing programs should only be conducted among high-risk groups

3.2.2   Recommended Regimens

Either individual antibiotics or combinations can be used [18, 19, 22, 23]. Isoniazid monotherapy has long been used, but combinations of isoniazid with rifampin or isoniazid with rifapentine allow for shorter duration of treatment. Rifampin alone can also be used. Efficacy of these regimens ranges from 60 to 90 % in adherent individuals [24, 25]. Protection is of variable duration and depends on the host (whether immunocompromised or not) and the risk of reexposure (community incidence). Recommended dosages for adults and for children are shown in Table 3.8. With regard to dosing frequency, daily regimens are generally used for isoniazid and for isoniazid plus rifampin. Isoniazid plus rifapentine is dosed once weekly for 12 weeks. Of note, the combination of rifampin plus pyrazinamide is *not* recommended and should be avoided because it has been associated with unacceptable rates of significant hepatotoxicity [26].

Isoniazid

Most commonly daily dosing for 6–9 months in low and moderate TB incidence settings is used. Efficacy is 60–90% in adherent individuals. In HIV-infected adults residing in settings of high TB transmission, at least 36 months of isoniazid is recommended as a proxy for lifelong treatment [21].

Combination of Isoniazid plus Rifapentine

Directly observed therapy is preferred since treatment is intermittently administered. It is well tolerated and associated with high treatment completion rates [27]. Compared to isoniazid alone, it has less hepatotoxicity but higher incidence of hypersensitivity (light headedness, dizziness, headache, nausea, vomiting, syncope, rash, or angioedema) and slightly higher rate of permanent discontinuation due to side effects, is well tolerated in children 2–17 years of age, and can also be

TABLE 3.8 Treatment for LTBI in adults and children

Drugs	Adult dose	Pediatric dose[a]
Isoniazid[b]	Standard regimen: 300 mg PO daily for 9 months Alternate regimens: 300 mg PO daily for 6 months 900 mg PO twice weekly for 9 months, given by DOT 900 mg PO twice weekly for 6 months, given by DOT	Standard regimen: 10–15 mg/kg PO daily for 9 months Maximum dose: 300 mg/day Alternate regimen: 20–30 mg/kg PO twice weekly for 9 months[c] Maximum dose: 900 mg/day

| Isoniazid plus Rifapentine | Isoniazid: PO once weekly for 12 doses, given by DOT
Dose is 15 mg/kg, rounded up to the nearest 50 or 100 mg; the typical dose is the maximal dose which is 900 mg
Rifapentine: PO once weekly for 12 doses, given by DOT. Typical adult dose is the maximal dose which is 900 mg. For adults << 50 kg, pediatric dosing can be used | Children ≥2 years and weighing at least 10 kg[d]
Isoniazid: PO once weekly for 12 doses, given by DOT
2–11 years: 25 mg/kg
≥12 years: 15 mg/kg
for both age groups the maximum weekly dose was 900 mg
Rifapentine: PO once weekly for 12 doses, given by DOT
10.0–14.0 kg: 300 mg
14.1–25.0 kg: 450 mg
25.1–32.0 kg: 600 mg
32.1–50.0 kg: 750 mg
>50.0 kg: 900 mg
Children who cannot swallow tablets can be administered a slurry of crushed INH and rifapentine tablets in either a soft food or liquid, starch based pudding (e.g., commercial chocolate pudding). Fruit-based carriers are discouraged |

(continued)

TABLE 3,8 (continued)

Drugs	Adult dose	Pediatric dose[a]
Rifampin	600 mg PO daily for 3–4 months	10–20 mg/kg PO daily for 4 months Maximum dose: 600 mg/day
Isoniazid plus Rifampin[e]	Isoniazid 300 mg PO daily for 3 months Rifampin 600 mg PO daily for 3 months	Isoniazid 10–15 mg/kg PO daily for 3 months Maximum dose: 300 mg/day Rifampin 10–20 mg/kg PO daily for 3 months Maximum dose: 600 mg/day

PO by mouth, *DOT* directly observed therapy

[a]Pediatric dose: <12 years

[b]Pyridoxine supplementation (25–50 mg PO daily for adults; 1–2 mg/kg PO daily for children <12) should be considered for patients on prolonged isoniazid; this is especially important for patients with conditions that can predispose to neuropathy (including diabetes, uremia, alcoholism, malnutrition and HIV infection), as well as in the setting of pregnancy and seizure disorders. In addition, pyridoxine should be administered to infants of breastfeeding mothers receiving isoniazid. Among children on isoniazid, pyridoxine is warranted for exclusively breastfed infants, children on meat- and milk-deficient diets, children with nutritional deficiencies, and symptomatic HIV-infected children

[c]Six-month regimens of isoniazid are not appropriate for children

[d]Dosing known for children 2 years and higher. Data from clinical trial NCT00023452 Villarino et al. [28]

[e]The regimen of isoniazid and rifampin is not recommended by the United States Centers for Disease Control and Prevention

used in HIV infected, but like rifampin, rifapentine has inter-actions with a number of other medications including many antiretrovirals and currently is only recommended with an efavirenz-based regimen (see Table 3.6). There are no data for pregnant or breastfeeding women. The main drawback for this regimen is the rifapentine drug-drug interactions.

Rifampin (Alone)

There are less data for rifampin alone, but efficacy appears to be similar to isoniazid monotherapy. Rifampin monotherapy is well tolerated with low rates of hepatotoxicity. Rifampin daily can be prescribed for 3 months or 4 months duration. This regimen is particularly useful for patients intolerant of isoniazid or for those with presumed infection with isoniazid-resistant *M. tuberculosis*. This regimen can also be used in children. There are limited data for pregnant women. The main drawback of rifampin monotherapy is that it has many drug-drug interactions (see Table 3.6).

Combination of Isoniazid plus Rifampin

Regimens containing both isoniazid plus rifampin should be considered for those likely exposed to isoniazid-resistant *M. tuberculosis*. Treatment with isoniazid plus rifampin is 3 or 4 months duration. This regimen can be used in children. There are limited data for use in pregnancy. The main drawback for this regimen is the rifampin drug-drug interactions.

Treatment of Multidrug-Resistant LTBI

The evidence base is insufficient as to the best treatment approach. Expert consultation should be sought, and manage-ment decisions should take into consideration a comprehensive individual risk-benefit assessment. Briefly, WHO recommends careful monitoring for at least 2 years after exposure to MDR-TB [20]. If the identity of the source case and the drug susceptibility profile of the source TB isolate are known with reasonable certainty, then an individually tailored regimen should be considered, but on the other hand if it is possible that the individual with LTBI was exposed to drug-susceptible TB, then a standard course of LTBI treatment should be considered. Treated individuals should be followed closely during and after (at least 18 months) treatment for medication side effects, breakthrough TB, and acquired resistance.

3.2.3   Practical Aspects

Selecting a Regimen

Selection of a regimen should take into consideration any comorbidities and concomitant medications, drug-drug interactions, any prior drug intolerance or adverse effect, adherence concerns, age, and whether pregnant or not. In places where rifapentine is available, the 3-month isoniazid plus rifapentine regimen, preferably with DOT, is an excellent alternative to 6–9 months of isoniazid.

Special Populations

   I. Persons who are intolerant of isoniazid or are presumed to have isoniazid mono-resistant infection: rifampin for 4 months can be used.

  II. Children <2 years: isoniazid or isoniazid plus rifampin can be considered.

III. Pregnant women: isoniazid for 6–9 months is currently the only regimen recommended for use in pregnancy. Initiation of isoniazid preventive therapy during pregnancy is recommended for women who are HIV infected or recently exposed to an active pulmonary TB case. There is increased hepatotoxicity risk during pregnancy and postpartum (usually within 3 months after delivery). There is a potential interaction between isoniazid and efavirenz. This interaction may or may not be clinically relevant in persons who are slow metabolizers of isoniazid and efavirenz.

IV. HIV infected: isoniazid, isoniazid plus rifampin, and isoniazid plus rifapentine have all been assessed in HIV-
infected individuals. As above, in resource-limited
settings with high TB incidence *and transmission*, treatment with isoniazid for 36 months or more (as a proxy for
lifelong) is recommended though adherence is a major
challenge, and this recommendation has been difficult to
implement. Neither rifampin nor rifapentine should be
used with protease inhibitors. The use of rifampin or rifapentine with integrase inhibitors requires dose adjustment (dose increase) of the integrase inhibitor. Other
drug interactions are shown in Table 3.5.

Adherence and Role of Directly Observed Therapy

Adherence to therapy is a critical determinant of clinical benefit. Therefore measures to facilitate adherence are desirable.
Direct observation of therapy as a means to facilitate adherence is preferred when intermittent LTBI regimens (e.g., 12
weeks of once-weekly isoniazid plus rifapentine) are used.

LTBI Patient Monitoring

The following five components comprise the monitoring plan
for patients on LTBI treatment.

I. Medical evaluation prior to LTBI treatment: obtaining a
thorough medical history is necessary before the initiation of LTBI treatment and serves several important func-
tions including building a rapport with the patient. The
initial evaluation should be used to review signs and
symptoms as a means of assessing for active TB disease;
inquire about the history of prior LTBI treatment or TB
disease, including any medication side effects; determine
if any other medical conditions are present that are associated with an increased risk of LTBI treatment side
effects or toxicity; review current and prior medications
for potential drug-drug interactions with LTBI treatment;
and recommend HIV testing and opt out screening.

Additionally, the benefits and potential side effects, as well as the importance of adherence to the treatment regimen and establishment of an optimal follow-up plan should be discussed during the initial medical evaluation.

Before LTBI treatment is prescribed, a chest radiograph is recommended to assess for active pulmonary TB.

For those patients with abnormalities on chest radiograph or with signs or symptoms concerning for possible active TB disease, preventive therapy should be deferred and the patient should promptly be evaluated for active TB disease. LTBI treatment should not be initiated until active TB disease has been reasonably excluded – typically this requires waiting several weeks for mycobacterial cultures to incubate.

II. Baseline laboratory testing: baseline laboratory testing is not routinely indicated for all patients at the start of treatment for LTBI. Baseline hepatic measurements of serum AST (SGOT) or ALT (SGPT) and bilirubin are indicated for individuals who have any of the following risk factors for hepatotoxicity: (1) signs of a liver disorder, (2) HIV infection, (3) are pregnant or at postpartum (within 3 months of delivery), (4) underlying liver disease (e.g., hepatitis B or C, alcoholic hepatitis, or cirrhosis), (5) consuming alcohol regularly, and (6) on other medications that are potentially hepatotoxic. For persons with liver chemistry elevations, the risks vs. benefits of LTBI treatment should be reassessed; many clinicians defer LTBI therapy (and seek an etiology of the liver chemistry elevations) if transaminases are ≥ 3 times the upper limit of normal.

III. Monthly evaluation: patients receiving LTBI treatment should be monitored at least monthly for adherence to the prescribed regimen, side effects or toxicity from the regimen, and signs and symptoms of TB disease. Patients should be educated to stop medication and seek medical attention promptly if any of the following symptoms of hepatitis are present: anorexia, nausea, vomiting, dark urine, icterus, rash, persistent paresthesias of the hands and feet, persistent fatigue, weakness or fever lasting three or more days, abdominal pain (particularly right upper quadrant discomfort), easy bruising or bleeding, or arthralgias. Patients receiving treatment by directly observed therapy should also be questioned at each dose about possible side effects.

IV. Routine laboratory monitoring: routine laboratory monitoring during treatment of LTBI is recommended for patients with any of the hepatotoxicity risk factors described above and also for patients with abnormal baseline liver function tests.

V. Management of liver side effects of LTBI treatment: LTBI treatment should immediately be discontinued when signs or symptoms of hepatitis develop, or when liver enzymes are five times the upper limit of normal in an asymptomatic person. The patient promptly should be evaluated clinically and with liver function testing. In patients with liver enzyme elevations that are less than five times the upper limit of normal and treatment is continued, close clinical and laboratory monitoring should be conducted.

VI. Treatment follow-up: at the treatment completion/follow-up visit, patients should be given documentation of their TST or IGRA results, TB medication taken, length of time on medication, and completion dates. They should present this information when they are required to be tested for TB. Patients should also be reeducated about the signs and symptoms of TB disease, advised to seek medical attention if these occur, and advised that treatment greatly reduces the risk of progression to disease, but does not entirely eliminate it.

Interrupted LTBI Therapy

Expert opinion recommends that in patients who have stopped taking their medications (6, 9, 12, or 36 months of isoniazid) for any reason, treatment can resume where it was left off if no more than 3 months were missed. If interruption has been more than 3 months, it is recommended to restart from the beginning. For shorter regimens of 2–4 months, patients missing more than 2 months should be reinitiated from the beginning.

Common Adverse Drug Reactions

See Table 3.5.

Drug-Drug Interactions

See Table 3.6.

References

1. Fox W, Ellard GA, Mitchison DA. Studies on the treatment of tuberculosis undertaken by the British Medical Research Council tuberculosis units, 1946–1986, with relevant subsequent publications. Int J Tuberc Lung Dis. 1999;3(10 Suppl 2):S231–79.
2. Iseman MD. A clinician's guide to tuberculosis. Philadelphia: Lippincott Williams & Wilkins; 2000.
3. Treatment of tuberculosis: guidelines – 4th ed. Geneva, World Health Organization, 2010 (WHO/HTM/TB/2009.420).
4. Zumla A, Nahid P, Cole ST. Advances in the development of new tuberculosis drugs and treatment regimens. Nat Rev Drug Discov. 2013;12(5):388–404.
5. Blumberg HM, Burman WJ, Chaisson RE, et al. American Thoracic Society/Centers for Disease Control and Prevention/Infectious Diseases Society of America: treatment of tuberculosis. Am J Respir Crit Care Med. 2003;167(4):603–62.
6. Benator D, Bhattacharya M, Bozeman L, et al. Rifapentine and isoniazid once a week versus rifampicin and isoniazid twice a week for treatment of drug-susceptible pulmonary tuberculosis in HIV-negative patients: a randomised clinical trial. Lancet. 2002;360(9332):528–34.
7. Jo KW, Yoo JW, Hong Y, et al. Risk factors for 1-year relapse of pulmonary tuberculosis treated with a 6-month daily regimen. Respir Med. 2014;108(4):654–9.
8. Lee CH, Wang WJ, Lan RS, Tsai YH, Chiang YC. Corticosteroids in the treatment of tuberculous pleurisy. A double-blind, placebo-controlled, randomized study. Chest. 1988;94(6):1256–9.
9. Galarza I, Canete C, Granados A, Estopa R, Manresa F. Randomised trial of corticosteroids in the treatment of tuberculous pleurisy. Thorax. 1995;50(12):1305–7.

10. Wyser C, Walzl G, Smedema JP, Swart F, van Schalkwyk EM, van de Wal BW. Corticosteroids in the treatment of tuberculous pleurisy. A double-blind, placebo-controlled, randomized study. Chest. 1996;110(2):333–8.

11. Elliott AM, Luzze H, Quigley MA, et al. A randomized, double-blind, placebo-controlled trial of the use of prednisolone as an adjunct to treatment in HIV-1-associated pleural tuberculosis. J Infect Dis. 2004;190(5):869–78.

12. Mayosi BM, Ntsekhe M, Bosch J, et al. Prednisolone and Mycobacterium indicus pranii in tuberculous pericarditis. N Engl J Med. 2014;371:1121–30.

13. Thwaites GE, Nguyen DB, Nguyen HD, et al. Dexamethasone for the treatment of tuberculous meningitis in adolescents and adults. N Engl J Med. 2004;351(17):1741–51.

14. Prasad K, Singh MB. Corticosteroids for managing tuberculous meningitis. Cochrane Database Syst Rev. 2008;1, CD002244.

15. Alsultan A, Peloquin CA. Therapeutic drug monitoring in the treatment of tuberculosis: an update. Drugs. 2014;74(8):839–54.

16. van Rie A, Warren R, Richardson M, et al. Exogenous reinfection as a cause of recurrent tuberculosis after curative treatment. N Engl J Med. 1999;341(16):1174–9.

17. Deciding when to treat latent TB infection. Available at http://www.cdc.gov/tb/topic/treatment/decideltbi.htm. Accessed 14 June 2016.

18. No authors listed. Targeted tuberculin testing and treatment of latent tuberculosis infection. Joint statement of the American Thoracic Society, and the Centers for Disease Control and Prevention. Am J Respir Crit Care Med. 2000;161(4 Pt 2):S221–47.

19. Getahun H, Matteelli A, Abubakar I, Abdel Aziz M, Baddeley A, et al. Management of latent Mycobacterium tuberculosis infection: WHO guidelines for low tuberculosis burden countries. Eur Respir J. 2015;46:1563–76.

20. World Health Organization. Guidelines on the management of latent tuberculosis infection. Geneva: World Health Organization; 2015 (WHO/HTM/TB/2015/01).

21. World Health Organization. Recommendations on 36 months isoniazid preventive therapy to adults and adolescents living with HIV in resource-constrained and high TB and HIV-prevalence settings: 2015 update. Geneva: World Health Organization; 2015 (WHO/HTM/TB/2015.15).

22. Centers for Disease Control and Prevention (CDC). Recommendations for use of an isoniazid-rifapentine regimen

with direct observation to treat latent Mycobacterium tuberculosis infection. MMWR Morb Mortal Wkly Rep. 2011;60:1650–3.

23. Treatment regimens for latent TB infection (LTBI). Available at http://www.cdc.gov/tb/topic/treatment/ltbi.htm. Accessed 14 June 2016.

24. Horsburgh Jr CR, Rubin EJ. Latent tuberculosis infection in the United States. N Engl J Med. 2011;364:1441–8.

25. Akolo C, Adetifa I, Shepperd S, Volmink J. Treatment of latent tuberculosis infection in HIV infected persons. Cochrane Database Syst Rev. 2010;1, CD000171.

26. Centers for Disease Control and Prevention (CDC); American Thoracic Society. Update: adverse event data and revised American Thoracic Society/CDC recommendations against the use of rifampin and pyrazinamide for treatment of latent tuberculosis infection – United States, 2003. MMWR Morb Mortal Wkly Rep. 2003;52:735–9.

27. Sterling TR, Villarino ME, Borisov AS, Shang N, Gordin F, et al. Three months of rifapentine and isoniazid for latent tuberculosis infection. N Engl J Med. 2011;365:2155–66.

28. Villarino ME, et al. Treatment for preventing tuberculosis in children and adolescents. JAMA Pediatr. 2015;169(3):247–55.

Chapter 4
Extrapulmonary Tuberculosis

Maunank Shah and Natasha Chida

4.1 Overview and Epidemiology

M. tuberculosis (MTB) can cause disease in almost any organ
of the body. Extrapulmonary tuberculosis (EPTB) is defined
as tuberculosis (TB) disease outside of the lung parenchyma
[1]. Much like pulmonary TB, EPTB can occur as a primary
infection or as reactivation of a latent focus with subsequent
spread. In primary infection the bacilli enter the body
through the lungs and then disseminate to other parts of the
body either via the lymphatic system or hematogenously;
alternatively a latent foci of bacilli may reactivate and then
disseminate in the same way. Globally, EPTB accounts for
approximately 15 % of new TB cases, but may be underre-

M. Shah (✉)
Department of Medicine, Division of Infectious Diseases, Johns
Hopkins University, Fisher Center, PCTB Room 224 N. Wolfe
St 725, Baltimore, MD 21205, USA
e-mail: mshah28@jhmi.edu

N. Chida
Department of Medicine, Division of Infectious Diseases, Johns
Hopkins University School of Medicine,
600 North Wolfe Street Phipps 540, Baltimore, MD 21287, USA
e-mail: nchida1@jhmi.edu

J.H. Grosset, R.E. Chaisson (eds.), *Handbook of Tuberculosis*, 91
DOI 10.1007/978-3-319-26273-4_4,
© Springer International Publishing Switzerland 2017

ported due to diagnostic challenges; many cases of EPTB continue to be diagnosed and treated based on clinical presentation and without microbiological confirmation [1]. The prevalence of EPTB among TB cases differs by geographic region, but may be affected by accuracy of reporting; for example, the World Health Organization (WHO) Eastern Mediterranean Region reports that 22 % of their total TB cases are EPTB in nature, while the Western Pacific region reports that 7 % of cases are EPTB [1].

The advent of the global HIV/AIDS epidemic has likely contributed to a rise in the worldwide burden of EPTB. Extrapulmonary or disseminated disease can be seen in more than 50 % of patients with concurrent HIV and TB as a consequence of immune suppression [2]. However, the HIV epidemic alone does not explain the observed increases in the proportion of EPTB in all countries. The United States (USA) is a high-income country with low overall HIV prevalence and low TB incidence, yet there has been a rise in the proportion of total TB cases attributable to EPTB. This observation has been attributed to a slower rate of decline of EPTB than pulmonary TB [3]. As such, the percent of TB cases in the United States that are EPTB has been increasing; in 2013 21 % of all TB cases were EPTB, compared to approximately 16 % in 1993 [3]. The underlying reasons for this evolving epidemiology remain unclear.

4.2   Overall Diagnosis and Treatment

The myriad presentations of EPTB create a significant challenge for clinicians. Symptoms are often specific to the organ system involved and may mimic more common disease conditions. Therefore, clinicians in endemic areas must maintain a high degree of suspicion for extrapulmonary forms of TB in order to avoid missing the diagnosis and should consider site-specific microbiological evaluations for MTB when assessments for common disease entities are unrevealing. As EPTB can occur anywhere in the body, symptoms of the disease may be related to the organ system or site involved. Systemic symptoms such as fevers, night sweats, and weight loss may be present, but are often nonspecific, fail to localize the disease, and do not alert clinicians to the underlying cause of illness.

The general approach to diagnosis of EPTB is similar to that for pulmonary TB. In patients with suspicion of EPTB involvement, biological specimens should be obtained from the affected tissue or fluid and sent for mycobacterial testing, including staining for acid fast bacilli (AFB), mycobacterial culture, and nucleic acid amplification testing (NAAT) when available. Histopathology can also be useful and may show characteristics consistent with TB disease such as necrotizing granulomas. Chest radiography (CXR) and sputum testing for AFB smear, culture, and NAAT are warranted to evaluate for concomitant pulmonary TB. Other indirect tests include tuberculin skin tests (TSTs), interferon gamma release assays (IGRAs), histopathology, chemistries and cell counts of body fluids, and radiologic studies. These indirect tests can provide additional data to lend support toward an EPTB diagnosis, but they should be interpreted with caution as they do not absolutely confirm or exclude TB as the underlying cause of disease presentation.

Given that presentations for EPTB can mimic serious disease conditions such as malignancy, fungal disease, or other bacterial infections, empiric TB therapy should be avoided when possible and a microbiological diagnosis should be aggressively pursued. Inappropriate EPTB diagnoses can lead to delays in diagnosis of other etiologies. Nonetheless, approximately 25–33 % of EPTB cases in areas with ready access to diagnostics, such as the United States and the European Union, continue to be diagnosed on the basis of clinical or radiographic suspicion; the global rate of empiric diagnosis is unclear, but is suspected to be higher [3, 4]. Among the reasons for this high percentage of clinical diagnoses is the poor sensitivity of current microbiological tests for EPTB. Mycobacterial culture is the most sensitive test available (i.e., ability to detect fewest number of bacilli) in extrapulmonary tissues/fluids, but is suboptimal; overall sensitivity ranges from 15 to 70 % depending on the site of TB disease [4, 5]. The emergence of nucleic acid amplification testing has increased the rapidity with which one can confirm a diagnosis of EPTB, but this technique has impaired diagnostic sensitivity; as such, a negative

NAAT test is usually insufficient to rule out EPTB disease. Nonetheless, the World Health Organization has published guidance on the usage of Xpert® MTB/RIF (Cepheid Inc., Sunnyvale, CA, USA), a rapid NAAT, for extrapulmonary TB diagnosis. Xpert MTB/RIF is now advocated as the preferred initial test of choice for evaluation of TB meningitis and can be used in place of usual practice for lymph nodes and other tissues in patients suspected of having EPTB [6]. However, mycobacterial cultures and additional microbiological testing should be concomitantly performed, particularly when Xpert MTB/RIF results do not identify MTB. In some patient populations, other emerging diagnostic assays may also be considered. Among HIV-infected individuals with advanced immunosuppression, urinary lipoarabinomannan (LAM) detection may be a strategy that allows for the detection of MTB, including extrapulmonary or disseminated forms of disease [7, 8]. The WHO has recently advocated the usage of the lateral-flow LAM (LF-LAM) assay for HIV-infected hospitalized individuals with CD4 < 100 or severe illness, a group with higher rates of disseminated disease (pooled sensitivity in meta-analyses of 56 %) [9].

The treatment of drug-susceptible EPTB depends on the site of disease. Many types of EPTB can be treated with the same standard therapy as that of pulmonary TB. This usually involves a total of 6 months of therapy and consists of 2 months of rifampin, isoniazid, pyrazinamide, and ethambutol (RHZE), followed by 4 months of rifampin and isoniazid (RH).

4.3   Specific Considerations

4.3.1   Pleural Tuberculosis

Pleural TB is one of the most frequent sites of EPTB infection, with some series reporting up to 20–37% of EPTB cases being pleural in nature [3, 4]. The pathophysiology of pleural TB is variable. In some cases it represents progression of primary disease from the lung parenchyma with direct extension to the pleural space; in others it is due to reactivation of latent disease in the pleural space, while in others it is due to disseminated disease. Pleural effusions are typically present and are more often unilateral than bilateral; they are thought to represent a hypersensitivity reaction to the bacilli within the pleural space [10, 11]. Patients may present with dyspnea, cough, pleuritic chest pain, and systemic symptoms, such as fevers and chills, or be asymptomatic.

The diagnosis of pleural TB is based upon radiographic appearance, evaluation of pleural fluid, and examination of pleural tissue. Pleural fluid is typically exudative, with lymphocytic predominance (though early in pleural TB pathogenesis, pleural fluid may demonstrate a neutrophilic predominance). Pleural fluid glucose and pH may be low or normal. Some experts have advocated adenosine deaminase (ADA) testing in pleural fluid, but sensitivity is low; nonetheless, a low ADA (<40 units per L) may have high negative predictive value in non-endemic settings [12, 13]. Of note, the sensitivity of AFB smear, mycobacterial culture, and NAAT is low in pleural fluid; mycobacterial culture positivity from pleural fluid is generally seen in less than 30 % of cases, although one series reported sensitivity as high as 70 % [14]. This low yield from pleural fluid may be the result of low bacillary load within the effusion. The sensitivity of Xpert MTB/RIF from pleural fluid has ranged from 0 to 100 %, with meta-analyses suggesting a pooled estimate of sensitivity of 17 % (95 % CI 7.5–34.2 %) when judged against a composite reference standard (but may be as high as 44 % [95 % CI 25–65 %] when judged against a culture reference standard). The specificity of Xpert MTB/RIF on pleural fluid is reported to be high (99 %, 95 % CI 94–100 %) [6].

Pleural tissue biopsy is the most sensitive microbiologic exam for the disease. Specimens should be sent for AFB smear, mycobacterial culture, and NAAT [15]. While culture remains the most sensitive diagnostic modality, the sensitivity of Xpert MTB/RIF on tissue has been reported in meta-analysis to be as high as 81 % (95 % CI 68–90 %) [6]. Histopathology of pleural tissue is also important; the presence of caseating granulomas on histopathology is highly suggestive of pleural TB. Lastly, some studies have found 20–59 % of pleural TB cases that occur with concurrent pulmonary TB; therefore, microbiologic examination of sputum samples is warranted [12].

The treatment of pleural TB focuses on medical management. The same 6-month standard drug regimen for drug-sensitive pulmonary disease is effective in the vast majority of pleural TB cases [16]. Currently, adjunctive steroids have not been recommended, though this has been debated in the literature. In two small randomized clinical trials, adjunctive steroid usage did not reduce the development of pleural thickening; alternatively some data has suggested a faster radiographic improvement with steroid usage, but the clinical importance of this finding is unknown [16–18].

The role of drainage for TB pleural effusions is less clear, but is currently advocated in the case of TB empyema, a form of pleural TB characterized by a large number of bacilli. This form of pleural TB is often the result of rupture of an adjacent pulmonary cavity, although occasionally a tuberculous pleural effusion can become an empyema. This form of pleural disease is usually characterized by a lower glucose than that of tuberculous pleural effusions (occasionally it can be less than 30 mg/dl) and a lower pH; they also tend to be more purulent in nature and to have a significant burden of bacilli [19, 20]. Occasionally, surgical interventions may be needed if pleural TB is complicated by bronchopleural fistulas.

4.3.2   Tuberculosis Lymphadenitis and Tuberculosis Abscess

TB lymphadenitis is among the most common extrapulmonary manifestations of TB, with 30–40 % EPTB cases being lymphatic in nature [3, 4]. It most often occurs in isolation, but can occur with concomitant pulmonary TB in 18–42 % of cases [21].

It is thought that most cases of TB lymphadenitis represent reactivation of bacilli that seeded the space previously, but disease due to disseminated primary infection can also occur [22]. While previously seen more commonly in children or young adults, HIV-coinfected patients and those with immunosuppression are also more likely to present with lymphatic forms of TB [21]. The cervical lymph node chain is among the most often affected and can lead to the classic presentation of "scrofula." However, TB lymphadenitis can occur at almost any body site: axillary, mesenteric, mediastinal, and inguinal TB lymphadenites are common sites of disease presentation. Nodes tend to be palpable when more superficially located and are often firm, discrete, and nontender. However, they may become matted in the case of multiple nodal involvement. If untreated, affected nodes may become fluctuant and abscess-like. If superficial, infected lymph nodes may begin to spontaneously drain and form a nonhealing sinus tract.

Tuberculous lymphadenitis is often a subacute or chronic process, which at times can distinguish it from other bacterial pathogens. Patients' only symptoms may be the presence of an enlarging node, although systemic symptoms such as fever and weight loss can occur. Diagnosis of TB lymphadenitis requires direct examination of the affected lymph node. Excisional biopsy offers the highest yield when sent for histopathology, AFB smear, mycobacterial culture, and NAAT; some studies report 80 % culture positivity [21]. A systematic review of Xpert MTB/RIF performed on lymph node tissue has suggested a diagnostic sensitivity of approximately 80 %, with high specificity (~99 %) when compared against a composite reference standard [6]. Fine needle aspiration is often performed in many clinical settings, but overall yield may be lower. In cases without a confirmed microbiological test from lymph node tissue, diagnosis is often based on excluding other etiologic considerations (including nontuberculous mycobacteria, fungal pathogens, bacterial pathogens, and malignancy).

Treatment of TB lymphadenitis or TB abscesses is focused on medical management with the standard TB drug regimens used for pulmonary TB for a 6-month duration [16]. While surgical interventions are often performed for diagnostic purposes, they are rarely required to cure TB lymphadenitis. However, for large and fluctuant nodes, drainage may be helpful [21, 23]. Incision and drainage are sometimes utilized for TB abscesses (e.g., psoas abscess), but data is limited comparing such approaches to medical management alone [24].

In the course of TB therapy, it is common for lymph nodes to enlarge. This "paradoxical" worsening does not usually indicate treatment failure, but rather an inflammatory reaction that results from the death of MTB bacilli. While there is limited data, minor inflammatory reactions can be managed with nonsteroidal anti-inflammatory drugs, and the use of steroids presumptively for TB lymphadenitis is not currently advocated [16, 21]. Some experts advocate the usage of steroids for severe inflammatory responses manifested by rapid nodal enlargement, extensive necrosis, or systemic symptoms such as fevers, but their efficacy in these settings is uncertain [25].

4.3.3   Central Nervous System (CNS) Tuberculosis

CNS TB consists of multiple manifestations including TB meningitis, intracranial tuberculoma, and tuberculous arachnoiditis. It is thought to occur most frequently as a result of early hematogenous dissemination during primary infection, but may represent reactivation of a latent focus of bacilli in patients without recent exposures [26].

CNS TB has been reported to occur in approximately 1 % of cases of TB worldwide, but has among the worst clinical outcomes [26]. In epidemiologic surveys of EPTB cases in the European Union and the United States, CNS TB represented 3.5 % and 5 % of EPTB cases, respectively [3, 4]. The mortality of TB meningitis has been found to be up to 65 % in some studies [26]. The risk of death and/or neurologic sequelae rises with therapeutic delays. CNS TB presents most commonly in children and in immunosuppressed individuals, including those with HIV infection. Patients often present in a subacute manner, initially with nonspecific systemic symptoms such as fevers and headache; occasionally personality changes can be seen. Eventually signs of meningitis, such as meningismus, worsened headache, focal neurological deficits, and altered mental status with progression to coma, may occur [26].

Brain imaging with CT or MRI may show basilar meningeal enhancement or hydrocephalus, which may occur due to obstruction of CSF flow. Lumbar puncture will typically reveal a low glucose concentration, elevated protein, and lymphocytic pleocytosis; however, early in the course of disease, cerebrospinal fluid (CSF) may have low numbers of leukocytes. The opening pressure is elevated in approximately 50 % of patients [26]. With regard to microbiological diagnosis, mycobacterial culture is the most sensitive available diagnostic modality, but remains imperfect and may take weeks to yield results. As such, the WHO has recommended Xpert MTB/RIF as the initial test of choice for TB meningitis, although mycobacterial culture should still be pursued if Xpert MTB/Rif is negative or if there is concern for MDR-TB [6]. The pooled estimate for sensitivity of Xpert MTB/RIF on CSF in meta-analyses has been reported to be approximately 80.5 % (when compared to a composite reference standard) with specificity of 97.8 %; a negative result does not rule out the diagnosis, but a positive result can be relied upon to guide initiation of therapy [5]. Given the lack of an ideal reference standard, evaluation of other body sites to confirm a microbiological diagnosis of TB should be pursued.

The differential diagnosis of TB meningitis is large and includes but is not limited to cryptococcal disease, other endemic fungal infections, neurosyphilis, herpes meningoencephalitis, melioidosis, brucellosis, and carcinomatous meningitis.

Tuberculomas represent foci of infection within the brain parenchyma. They may be asymptomatic or produce focal neurological deficits that correlate to the location of the lesion. Tuberculomas may also obstruct CSF pathways, leading to increased intracranial pressure. On brain imaging such lesions may have peripheral edema and ring enhancement, although early-stage disease can lack these features. In the appropriate setting, neurocysticercosis and toxoplasmosis should be considered in the differential diagnosis of tuberculoma. Definitive diagnoses can be made via tissue biopsy, but given the morbidity of such a procedure, the diagnosis is often made empirically in the setting of systemic signs and symptoms of TB.

Spinal tuberculous arachnoiditis is a focal TB disease of the spinal cord. It may be clinically silent and subacute or may present with meningitis-like symptoms. Focal neurological deficits may occur and will correlate to the location of disease. Cord compression may also occur, as well as thrombosis of the spinal vasculature with resulting spinal cord infarction. MRI is useful in considering spinal tuberculous arachnoiditis, but tissue biopsy for AFB smear, mycobacterial culture, and NAAT testing is required to make a diagnosis.

Current guidelines recommend a total of 9–12 months of therapy for CNS TB; this usually consists of 2 months of RHZE, followed by 7–10 months of RH [16]. However, due to the fact that ethambutol penetrates poorly into the CNS, there is growing interest in evaluating alternate agents. The WHO recommends replacing ethambutol with streptomycin, although the use of aminoglycosides is not without difficulty; therefore there is interest in exploring the use of fluoroquinolones and other agents in TB meningitis [23, 26, 27]. In addition, there is also data that increasing the dose of rifampin (and parenteral administration) for patients with TB meningitis may lead to improved outcomes, although current guidelines do not reflect this [28]. Of note, tuberculomas may enlarge while patients are on antituberculous therapy; such enlargement is not necessarily indicative of treatment failure and may be due to inflammatory responses.

The use of corticosteroids for TB meningitis has been shown to reduce mortality in HIV-uninfected patients by approximately 30 % and also residual neurological deficits; however, it appears the benefit of steroids decreases with advanced disease [29]. Current recommendations advocate administration of steroids to patients with TB meningitis, though the optimal dose and duration are less clear [16, 23].

Due to the risk of immune reconstitution inflammatory syndrome (IRIS) with antiretroviral therapy (ART) initiation among HIV-infected individuals, the question of when to start ART in HIV patients with TB meningitis has been one of great interest. One trial in Vietnam found that immediate ART initiation was not associated with increased mortality, but adverse events were increased [30]. Current general guidelines recommend ART initiation within 2–4 weeks of antituberculous therapy in patients with CD4 counts of less than 50, and ART initiation within 2–3 months of therapy for patients with CD4 counts great than 50 [31], but caution should be exercised in patients with TB meningitis. Some experts recommend deferring ART initiation in TB meningitis regardless of CD4 count until patients have received at least 2 months of therapy [30].

4.3.4   Ocular Tuberculosis

Ocular TB can occur within the eye or involve the extraocular structures of the eye. The reported prevalence of ocular TB among TB cases has varied from <1 % to 18 % in epidemiologic studies [32, 33]. Such data is difficult to interpret, as many diagnoses of ocular TB are made on clinical grounds alone without microbiological confirmation. Orbital TB can occur from hematogenous spread or extension from contiguous structures [34].

Intraocular TB most often presents as granulomatous uveitis affecting the iris and ciliary body (anterior uveitis) or the choroidal body (posterior uveitis). It is thought that posterior uveitis is the most common presentation of intraocular TB [35]. Patients may present with visual changes and eye pain. In such cases microbiological diagnosis is often difficult to obtain; physical examination combined with systemic findings of active or latent TB is often used to make a diagnosis of intraocular TB [32]. On ophthalmologic examination choroidal granulomas, retinal vasculitis, choroidal tubercles, choroiditis, and endophthalmitis may be seen [35]. Retinal TB without posterior uveitis can occur but is uncommon. The differential diagnosis of uveitis includes herpes simplex infection, syphilis infection, sarcoidosis, and fungal infections.

Symptoms of extraocular TB depend on the structure involved and may include blurred vision, eye pain, and complete loss of vision. Diagnosis may be made via sampling of the tissue from the affected site for AFB smear, mycobacterial culture, and NAAT; the sensitivity of diagnostic testing varies based on the type of tissue being sampled (glandular, bone, etc.). Histopathology may show caseating granulomas. Scleral TB is rare, and due to sampling difficulties, the diagnosis is often made via physical examination and evidence of systemic active or latent TB infection [34].

Current guidelines do not offer specific treatment plans for extraocular or ocular TB, but most experts recommend a standard 6-month drug regimen. Extended duration can be considered if there is concomitant CNS disease or for slow clinical improvement. If intraocular TB is suspected, topical steroids or low-dose oral steroids are often added until a clinical response is seen.

4.3.5   Pericardial Tuberculosis

In many endemic settings, TB is the most common etiologic agent causing pericarditis [36, 37]. TB pericarditis can develop due to contiguous spread from adjacent structures (mediastinal nodes, lung tissue, or spine), as a result of dissemination to the pericardium (as is seen in cases of miliary TB) or, less commonly, as a result of reactivation in pericardial tissue [37]. Prompt diagnosis and treatment are required to avoid adverse outcomes. Globally, mortality associated with TB pericarditis is as high as 26 %, and even higher among those with HIV coinfection [38]. Clinical features are consistent with pericarditis and can include chest pain, dyspnea, and tamponade physiology when severe; fever and cough may also be seen. A clue to the diagnosis in low-prevalence areas is the persistence of effusion over time and lack of resolution with nonsteroidal anti-inflammatory agents.

Diagnosis of TB pericarditis can be challenging owing to the difficulties of obtaining adequate tissue and fluid for microbiological testing and the imperfect sensitivity of the reference standard test (i.e., mycobacterial culture). As 10–55 % of cases may have concomitant pulmonary TB, evaluating sputum for

AFB smear, mycobacterial culture, and NAAT testing should be considered [37, 39, 40].

Pericardiocentesis is indicated whenever TB pericarditis is suspected; fluid should be sent for fluid analysis (including a cell count and protein), AFB smear, and mycobacterial culture. The use of NAATs such as the Xpert MTB/RIF on pericardial fluid has not been studied widely at this time. Like pleural fluid, tuberculous pericardial effusions are often exudative; fluid may be bloody and usually have a high protein count and increased leukocyte count with lymphocytosis [37]. The culture of pericardial fluid yields a diagnosis in only 50–75 % of cases; therefore, a negative culture does not rule out the disease [41, 42]. ADA testing on the pericardial fluid may be helpful, although the optimal cutoff value to define positivity for this test has not been determined, and sensitivity and specificity therefore vary in current literature [43].

When culture of pericardial fluid fails to yield a diagnosis, or there is no pericardial fluid to obtain, a biopsy of pericardial tissue may be required. This is particularly true in low-prevalence settings where other causes of persistent pericarditis (such as malignancy, sarcoidosis, or rheumatologic processes) are more common. Although results are conflicting, culture of pericardial tissue seems to have a higher yield than pericardial fluid culture, with some small studies finding positivity of up to 70–100 % [44–46]. NAAT testing of pericardial tissue should also be considered, and tissue pathology may show caseating granulomas.

The treatment of TB pericarditis includes standard therapy with RHZE for 2 months followed by RH for 4 months, with close monitoring for complications of constrictive pericarditis [16]. Current guidelines advocate the addition of glucocorticoids for the first 11 weeks of therapy on the basis of several small studies suggesting possible reduced mortality and reduced need for pericardiocentesis. However, the role of corticosteroids for TB pericarditis has recently come under scrutiny. In 2009 a Cochrane review of interventions to treat pericarditis examined the question of steroids and did not find a statistically significant reduction in mortality among patients who received them. Subsequently, in 2014 the largest randomized trial evaluating the use of steroids in TB pericarditis was published [38]. 1400 adults with confirmed or probable pericardial TB were randomized to receive prednisolone or placebo; there was no improvement in the primary composite outcome of death, tamponade, or constrictive pericarditis among those that received prednisolone compared to placebo (HR 0.95 95 % CI 0.77–1.18). In secondary analysis of specific outcomes, prednisolone usage was associated with reduced hazard of constrictive pericarditis (HR 0.56 95 % CI 0.36–0.87) and hospitalizations (HR 0.79 85 % CI 0.63–0.99). However, there was also an increase in cancer among those in the prednisolone arm largely driven by HIV-associated malignancies. The optimal duration and dosage of steroid usage in pericardial TB thus remain unclear.

4.3.6   Skeletal Tuberculosis

Currently bone and joint TB appears to account for up to 11 % of EPTB cases based on the US and European surveillance data, but may account for up to 20 % of cases in other regions [3, 4, 47]. The development of skeletal TB can occur as a result of hematogenous seeding during primary disease or during reactivation of a previously seeded site. Spinal TB involving thoracic vertebral bodies (also known as Pott's disease) is the most common skeletal manifestation of TB, occurring in up to 50 % of skeletal TB cases [48]. It typically manifests with infection of the anterior portion of the vertebral body of the lower thoracic and upper lumbar spine, with subsequent destruction of the intervertebral disk space (although this occurs later in the disease, early on disk sparing may be seen). Radiographically, anterior wedging can be seen on CT or MRI. Paraspinal (or psoas) abscesses are often seen in conjunction with skeletal TB. The second most common site of skeletal TB is tuberculous arthritis and then extraspinal osteomyelitis [47].

The main clue for clinicians of spinal TB is pain at the site of infection that is chronic and progressive. Given the lack of specificity of the clinical syndrome, clinicians must have a high index of suspicion for the skeletal TB, particularly in endemic areas. Systemic symptoms such as fever and weight loss may be present, but this is not uniform. In TB arthritis, joint effusion and edema develop slowly, and typical signs of joint infection, such as warmth and erythema, may be absent [49]. Delayed diagnosis of vertebral TB can lead to cord compression, while joint destruction with loss of function can be a consequence of TB arthritis.

Like the other types of EPTB, the diagnosis of skeletal TB rests on obtaining a sample for AFB smear, mycobacterial culture, and NAAT of the affected site. When the disease is suspected, biopsy should be pursued of the bone or synovial tissue (depending on the site affected). Culture positivity on the bone and synovial tissue is between 35 and 48 %, while caseating granulomas may be seen on pathology [6]. Joint effusion fluid can be analyzed but may not be inflammatory in nature [50]. In one series the mean leukocyte count of TB-related joint effusions was approximately 15,000; either a neutrophilic or lymphocytic predominance may be seen [50]. The yield of culture of joint effusions is low, with some studies reporting positivity rates of less than 20 % [50]. Xpert MTB/RIF should be obtained on tissue specimens and appears to have a sensitivity of up to 82 % on the bone compared to a composite reference sample; however, its use in joint fluid has not been fully studied and is not currently recommended [6].

Current data suggests that 6–12 months of antituberculous therapy (initial 2-month intensive phase with RHZE, followed by 4–10 months of RH) is as effective as 18 months of therapy without rifamycins [16]. Most clinical experts and guidelines favor 6–9 months of therapy using first-line drugs, with therapy sometimes being extended to 12 months for severe cases or Pott's disease [16, 51]. Adjunctive surgical management can be considered on a case-by-case basis for the management of treatment failure, progression of lesions, cord compression, or joint instability. To date, data is insufficient to support routine adjunctive surgical management compared to medical chemotherapy alone. The role of newer antituberculous agents with improved bone and joint penetration in the management of skeletal TB (such as fluoroquinolones) is unknown.

4.3.7   Genitourinary Tuberculosis

Genitourinary (GU) TB disease refers to TB disease anywhere in the genitourinary tract, including the renal parenchyma. GU TB comprises 6–7 % of EPTB cases based on the US and European epidemiologic data, but has been reported to represent up to 40 % of EPTB cases in specific regions [3, 4]. It is thought that most cases of GU TB result from hematogenous dissemination during primary infection. Dysuria, hematuria, sterile pyuria, and/or flank pain is common clinical symptoms associated with renal TB, though renal function is usually preserved and patients may be asymptomatic [52, 53]. Testicular TB can present with testicular enlargement that is often misdiagnosed as testicular cancer on the basis of symptomatology and radiographic appearance. Ovarian or fallopian tube TB often goes unrecognized until lesions become large and can be asymptomatic; involvement of the female reproductive tract is often first recognized in the process of fertility evaluation in women of reproductive age.

Diagnosis of GU TB often requires radiographic imaging, in addition to microbiological testing of urine and tissue. Imaging may reveal renal abscesses or calcifications, ureteral strictures, thickened or contracted bladder, tubo-ovarian abscesses, and/or enlarged testes. Genital involvement often occurs with concurrent renal TB, and urinary testing for AFB smear, culture, and NAAT along with renal/tissue biopsy can be considered. The range of culture positivity varies across studies, from 11 to 80 % [53]; the sensitivity of urine mycobacterial culture may increase with additional samples. Rates of culture positivity on renal/GU tissue are not well defined, but are likely to be similar to that of other tissues. The use of Xpert MTB/RIF on urine has not been fully studied and is not currently recommended, but one validation study of Xpert

MTB/RIF reported a sensitivity of up to 100 % compared to a composite reference standard [54].

For the treatment of GU TB, a standard 6-month antituberculous regimen is recommended, and responses are favorable [16]. In some cases of large renal or tubo-ovarian abscesses, adjunctive drainage or surgery can be considered, but such procedures are generally reserved for severe cases. When complicated by ureteral obstructions/strictures with hydronephrosis, nephrostomy tubes may be required.

4.3.8   Gastrointestinal Tuberculosis

Gastrointestinal (GI) TB comprises 3–5 % of EPTB cases in the US and European epidemiologic data and may be more prevalent in other parts of the world; some studies have reported up to 16 % of TB cases having abdominal involvement [3, 4, 55]. Gastrointestinal and abdominal TB can have diverse manifestations. The ileocecal or ileojejunal areas are common sites of disease, although any part of the GI tract can be affected. It is thought that GI TB arises from either swallowing the bacilli in infected sputum or contaminated food, hematogenous spread, or contiguous spread of disease [56]. Abdominal pain, diarrhea, gastric outlet obstruction, perforation, melena, and rectal bleeding are all possible presentations, with or without systemic symptoms; ulcers within the GI tract may also occur [57]. The differential diagnosis of GI TB often includes Crohn's disease, ulcerative colitis, and malignancy. It is important to distinguish these entities through histopathology of affected tissue in conjunction with microbiological testing. In endemic settings, GI TB is often misdiagnosed or missed while evaluating for inflammatory bowel disease. Imaging via computed tomography (CT) scan of the abdomen may be helpful to assess both the extent of disease and potential etiology.

Peritoneal TB is another manifestation of GI TB that can occur as a result of reactivation of bacilli in the peritoneal space or mesenteric lymph nodes. Patients may present with subacute symptoms of abdominal pain and swelling and with systemic symptoms such as weight loss, loss of appetite, and fever. Ascites occurs in approximately 80 % of patients [58]. Evaluation of ascites fluid often shows elevated proteins of >3.0 g/dl and, in the absence of concomitant cirrhosis, a low serum/ascites albumin gradient of less than 1.1 [59]. Cell counts of the fluid reveal a lymphocytic-predominant cell count, although the range of leukocytes is variable [58]. Liver involvement can present with single or multiple abscesses and is often associated with disseminated disease.

Mycobacterial culture of stool and gastric fluid should be performed when suspecting TB within the GI tract lumen, but the sensitivity of these tests appears to be low [55, 56]. It should also be noted that isolation of TB from gastric lavage fluid may indicate pulmonary TB (and swallowed sputa), rather than GI involvement. Xpert MTB/RIF has been evaluated for use in gastric fluids; the pooled estimate for sensitivity of Xpert from gastric lavage compared against culture is 84 % (95 % CI 66–93 %), but is dependent on good quality samples and the degree of upper GI involvement [6]. In addition, the yield of Xpert MTB/RIF in stool specimens is being evaluated. In one study patients with and without pulmonary TB underwent Xpert MTB/RIF fecal testing; the sensitivity in stool specimens was 100 % in patients with 1+–3+ smear-positive disease, 81 % for patients with scant smear positivity, and 50 % for smear-negative patients [60]. If noninvasive testing does not yield a diagnosis, endoscopy or colonoscopy may be required to obtain tissue for AFB smear, mycobacterial culture, NAAT, and histopathology. The yield of culture is unknown in these specimens, but appears to be low based on the results of small studies [57]. Pathology may show caseating granulomas.

For extraintestinal forms of GI or abdominal TB, diagnostic sampling of affected tissue (peritoneal biopsy, ascites, and liver biopsy) should be performed and samples sent for histopathology, AFB smear and culture, and NAAT when available. The yield of culture of ascitic fluid is low, with some series reporting culture positivity rates of 9–20 %, while the yield of peritoneal biopsy mycobacterial culture is not clearly defined [58, 61]. Histopathology may show granulomas [58, 59]. The use of Xpert MTB/RIF in peritoneal fluid has not been fully evaluated, but one small study that included peritoneal specimens in a category of "body fluid" found an overall sensitivity of 86–100 % compared to a composite reference standard; however, studies specifically evaluating peritoneal fluid are needed [62]. ADA with a cutoff value of 39 IU/L has also been proposed for use in ascites fluid, but the sensitivity of this test varies in patients with cirrhosis [63]. In addition, given that up to 20 % of patients with GI TB have concomitant pulmonary TB, an evaluation of sputum for AFB smear, mycobacterial culture, and NAAT can be considered [57].

The treatment of both GI and peritoneal TB consists of standard 6-month antituberculous regimen [16]. Concomitant use of steroids is not recommended; in one small study, patients who received steroids for peritoneal TB had less fibrotic complications than those who did not, but the difference was not statistically significant [16]. Regarding intraluminal GI TB, if bowel obstruction, perforation, strictures, or bleeding is present, a surgical evaluation may be required.

4.3.9 Cutaneous Tuberculosis

Cutaneous TB is rare and is estimated to occur in 1–2 % of EPTB cases [64, 65]. The presentations of cutaneous TB are varied and classified based on the mechanisms of entry to the cutaneous tissue, along with the host's immunological status; the pathophysiology of the disease also depends on these variables. Cutaneous TB can result from exogenous inoculation, endogenous spread, and hematogenous spread [65, 66].

Exogenous inoculation, most common in laboratory workers, can lead to a tuberculosis chancre (TC), tuberculosis verrucosa cutis (TVC), or lupus vulgaris (LV) [64]. It is hypothesized that patients develop either TC or TVC depending on whether they have been previously infected and sensitized to the organism previously. TC is associated with primary inoculation in an unsensitized patient; after inoculation reddish-brown papules develop over several weeks, with eventual ulceration. Lesions are usually less than 1 cm in diameter and may include adjacent lymphadenopathy and granulomatous inflammation on biopsy. There is felt to be greater bacillary replication and load in TC, and MTB can often be isolated if mycobacterial culture of the lesion is performed; immunologic assays such as TST or IGRA may be negative initially. By contrast, TVC usually occurs after inoculation into the skin of a patient with prior sensitization; it is often characterized by few bacilli and acute neutrophilic infiltrates on biopsy. Culture is often negative with TVC, while immunologic assays such as TST or IGRA are often positive. Clinically TVC may present with lesions 1–5 cm in diameter and be violaceous brown and verrucous in nature with an atrophic center; spontaneous healing may occur over months to years. While lupus vulgaris usually originates from endogenous TB with hematogenous spread, it can also be the result of direct inoculation and tends to be paucibacillary; mycobacterial culture is therefore often negative [64]. There are multiple clinical variants of LV with manifestations ranging from plaquelike forms to nodular or tumorlike forms; multiple lesions can occur and coalesce and resolution without treatment is less common.

Secondary forms of cutaneous TB occur from hematogenous or contiguous spread and are more common than TC or TVC [65]. Scrofuloderma is a unique form of cutaneous TB due to reactivation of TB from contiguous tissue (usually lymph node or bone) or contiguous spread of primary infection from an underlying structure [67]. The lesions usually begin as subcutaneous nodules with progressive liquefaction and generation of a cold abscess and sinus tract. The disease is multibacillary and culture is often positive. Hematogenous spread to cutaneous tissues can be seen in patients with disseminated or miliary TB and also tends to be multibacillary; skin lesions are often discrete pin-sized red or blue papules that eventually form scars. TB gumma (tuberculous abscess) is also possible in patients with hematogenous spread and presents as a subcutaneous abscess, which often breaks down to form a nonhealing sinus tract.

Finally, "tuberculids" are cutaneous manifestations believed to be immunologically mediated and without direct microbial involvement of cutaneous tissues [67]. Mycobacterial culture is therefore rarely positive. Papulonecrotic tuberculids are recurrent crops of reddish papules often on the buttocks; histopathology will show wedge-shaped necrosis of the upper dermis on histopathology. Erythema induratum ("of Bazin") is a form of tuberculid characterized by a nodular vasculitis with areas of fat necrosis and lobular panniculitis. Its relationship to MTB has been debated in the literature, though some case reports have isolated MTB nucleic acid using PCR [65].

The diagnosis of cutaneous TB can be challenging and involves mycobacterial culture of tissue, immunologic testing to evaluate for prior TB infection (through TST and/or IGRA), and histopathology; however, the yield of these tests depends on whether the cutaneous form of TB present is multibacillary or paucibacillary. Treatment is aimed at eradicating underlying replicating bacilli and sterilizing any metabolically inactive forms of TB (similar to pulmonary TB treatment approaches).

The bacillary load in many forms of cutaneous TB may be low, raising the questions of what an appropriate regimen for cutaneous TB is and what the duration of treatment should be. Nonetheless, current approaches favor conservative treatment to include 6 months of standard antituberculosis drugs consistent with the regimens recommended for pulmonary TB [51].

4.3.10   Miliary Tuberculosis

Miliary TB occurs when a focus of MTB infiltrates into a vascular or lymphatic channel, spreads via a hematogenous or lymphatic route, and results in diffuse tubercles; tubercles can occur in any organ of the body [68]. The disease may occur during primary infection or during reactivation of latent TB.

The epidemiology of miliary TB is not well defined, likely due to difficulties in diagnosis. Globally it is estimated that 1–2 % of current TB cases among immunocompetent patients are miliary in nature [68]. In the United States, the proportion of miliary TB among all reported TB cases has increased from 1.3 % in the late 1980s to 3.7 % in 2013 [69, 70]. Immune suppression is considered a risk factor for the development of disseminated disease; very young children and the elderly are also at risk, presumably because of diminished T-cell responses. The HIV epidemic, rising prevalence of diabetes mellitus, aging of the global population, and increased use of TNF-alpha inhibitors for rheumatologic diseases may account for some of the increase in miliary TB. In one series, 4.6–6.6 % of patients with HIV and TB coinfection had either miliary TB or TB in more than two organs [2].

Patients with miliary TB may additionally have TB mycobacteremia (though the two conditions can occur independently as well) and may present with nonspecific systemic symptoms such as fever, night sweats, and weight loss. Alternatively, patients may have acute and severe disease presentations with manifestations of septic shock. Clinicians must therefore maintain a high level of suspicion for these disseminated forms of disease, particularly given that mortality associated with miliary disease or mycobacteremia in adults is estimated to be 25–30 % [68]. A successful diagnosis depends on obtaining imaging and microbiologic data from sites suspected to be involved. At least 50 % of patients with miliary TB have pulmonary involvement; therefore, an evaluation for pulmonary disease should be undertaken with chest imaging and sputum for AFB smear, culture, and NAAT testing [68, 71]. However, negative testing for pulmonary TB does not exclude a diagnosis of miliary TB, as the bacilli may be primarily located in the lymphatics and not the lung parenchyma. Mycobacterial blood cultures can be obtained to evaluate for the presence of mycobacteremia. Given that 10–30 % of patients with disseminated disease in some settings may have concomitant TB meningitis, lumbar puncture can be considered if patients exhibit signs and symptoms concerning CNS disease [68].

The treatment of miliary TB disease includes 6 months of standard antituberculosis drugs (provided that TB meningitis or bony involvement is not present) [16].

References

1. World Health Organization. Global tuberculosis report, 2014. 2014. Available at: http://www.who.int/tb/publications/global_report/en/. Accessed 1 Feb 2015.
2. Manosuthi W, Chottanapand S, Thongyen S, Chaovavanich A, Sungkanuparph S. Survival rate and risk factors of mortality among HIV/tuberculosis-coinfected patients with and without antiretroviral therapy. J Acquir Immune Defic Syndr. 2006;43(1): 42–6.
3. Peto HM, Pratt RH, Harrington TA, LoBue PA, Armstrong LR. Epidemiology of extrapulmonary tuberculosis in the United States, 1993–2006. Clin Infect Dis. 2009;49(9):1350–7.
4. Sandgren A, Hollo V, van der Werf MJ. Extrapulmonary tuberculosis in the European Union and European Economic Area, 2002 to 2011. Euro Surveill. 2013;18(12):20431.
5. Denkinger CM, Schumacher SG, Boehme CC, Dendukuri N, Pai M, Steingart KR. Xpert MTB/RIF assay for the diagnosis of extrapulmonary tuberculosis: a systematic review and meta-analysis. Eur Respir J. 2014;44(2):435–46.
6. World Health Organization. Xpert MTB/RIF: WHO Policy update and Implementation manual. 2013. Available at: http://www.who.int/tb/laboratory/xpert_launchupdate/en/. Accessed 1 Feb 2015.
7. Lawn SD, Dheda K, Kerkhoff AD, Peter JG, Dorman S, Boehme CC, et al. Determine TB-LAM lateral flow urine antigen assay for HIV-associated tuberculosis: recommendations on the design and reporting of clinical studies. BMC Infect Dis. 2013;13:407-2334-13-407.
8. Shah M, Martinson NA, Chaisson RE, Martin DJ, Variava E, Dorman SE. Quantitative analysis of a urine-based assay for detection of lipoarabinomannan in patients with tuberculosis. J Clin Microbiol. 2010;48(8):2972–4.
9. World Health Organization. The use of lateral flow LAM for the diagnosis and screening of active TB in people living with HIV. 2015. Available at: http://www.who.int/tb/publications/use-of-lf-lam-tb-hiv/en/. Accessed 1 Feb 2015.

10. Cases Viedma E, Lorenzo Dus MJ, Gonzalez-Molina A, Sanchis Aldas JL. A study of loculated tuberculous pleural effusions treated with intrapleural urokinase. Respir Med. 2006;100(11): 2037–42.

11. Light R. Pleural diseases. 5th ed. Philadelphia: Williams & Wilkins; 2007. p. 211–24.

12. Kim HJ, Lee HJ, Kwon SY, Yoon HI, Chung HS, Lee CT, et al. The prevalence of pulmonary parenchymal tuberculosis in patients with tuberculous pleuritis. Chest. 2006;129(5):1253–8.

13. McGrath EE, Anderson PB. Diagnostic tests for tuberculous pleural effusion. Eur J Clin Microbiol Infect Dis. 2010; 29(10):1187–93.

14. Valdes L, Alvarez D, San Jose E, Penela P, Valle JM, Garcia-Pazos JM, et al. Tuberculous pleurisy: a study of 254 patients. Arch Intern Med. 1998;158(18):2017–21.

15. Gopi A, Madhavan SM, Sharma SK, Sahn SA. Diagnosis and treatment of tuberculous pleural effusion in 2006. Chest. 2007;131(3):880–9.

16. Blumberg HM, Burman WJ, Chaisson RE, Daley CL, Etkind SC, Friedman LN, et al. American Thoracic Society/Centers for Disease Control and Prevention/Infectious Diseases Society of America: treatment of tuberculosis. Am J Respir Crit Care Med. 2003;167(4):603–62.

17. Wyser C, Walzl G, Smedema JP, Swart F, van Schalkwyk EM, van de Wal BW. Corticosteroids in the treatment of tuberculous pleurisy. A double-blind, placebo-controlled, randomized study. Chest. 1996;110(2):333–8.

18. Lee CH, Wang WJ, Lan RS, Tsai YH, Chiang YC. Corticosteroids in the treatment of tuberculous pleurisy. A double-blind, placebo-controlled, randomized study. Chest. 1988;94(6):1256–9.

19. Sahn SA, Iseman MD. Tuberculous empyema. Semin Respir Infect. 1999;14(1):82–7.

20. Berger HW, Mejia E. Tuberculous pleurisy. Chest. 1973;63(1): 88–92.

21. Fontanilla JM, Barnes A, von Reyn CF. Current diagnosis and management of peripheral tuberculous lymphadenitis. Clin Infect Dis. 2011;53(6):555–62.

22. Alvarez S, McCabe WR. Extrapulmonary tuberculosis revisited: a review of experience at Boston City and other hospitals. Medicine (Baltimore). 1984;63(1):25–55.

23. World Health Organization. Guidelines for treatment of tuberculosis. 2010. Available at: http://www.who.int/tb/publications/2010/9789241547833/en/. Accessed 1 Feb 2015.

24. Harrigan RA, Kauffman FH, Love MB. Tuberculous psoas abscess. J Emerg Med. 1995;13(4):493–8.
25. Hawkey CR, Yap T, Pereira J, Moore DA, Davidson RN, Pasvol G, et al. Characterization and management of paradoxical upgrading reactions in HIV-uninfected patients with lymph node tuberculosis. Clin Infect Dis. 2005;40(9):1368–71.
26. Thwaites GE, van Toorn R, Schoeman J. Tuberculous meningitis: more questions, still too few answers. Lancet Neurol. 2013;12(10):999–1010.
27. Torok ME. Tuberculous meningitis: advances in diagnosis and treatment. Br Med Bull. 2015;113(1):117–31.
28. Ruslami R, Ganiem AR, Dian S, Apriani L, Achmad TH, van der Ven AJ, et al. Intensified regimen containing rifampicin and moxifloxacin for tuberculous meningitis: an open-label, randomised controlled phase 2 trial. Lancet Infect Dis. 2013;13(1):27–35.
29. Prasad K, Singh MB. Corticosteroids for managing tuberculous meningitis. Cochrane Database Syst Rev. 2008;(1):CD002244.
30. Torok ME, Yen NT, Chau TT, Mai NT, Phu NH, Mai PP, et al. Timing of initiation of antiretroviral therapy in human immunodeficiency virus (HIV)--associated tuberculous meningitis. Clin Infect Dis. 2011;52(11):1374–83.
31. United States Department of Health and Human Services. Guidelines for the use of antiretroviral agents in HIV-1-infected adults and adolescents. 2015. Available at: http://aidsinfo.nih.gov/ guidelines. Accessed 1 June 2015.
32. Thompson MJ, Albert DM. Ocular tuberculosis. Arch Ophthalmol. 2005;123(6):844–9.
33. Alvarez GG, Roth VR, Hodge W. Ocular tuberculosis: diagnostic and treatment challenges. Int J Infect Dis. 2009;13(4):432–5.
34. Madge SN, Prabhakaran VC, Shome D, Kim U, Honavar S, Selva D. Orbital tuberculosis: a review of the literature. Orbit. 2008; 27(4):267–77.
35. Abu El-Asrar AM, Abouammoh M, Al-Mezaine HS. Tuberculous uveitis. Int Ophthalmol Clin. 2010;50(2):19–39.
36. Cherian G. Diagnosis of tuberculous aetiology in pericardial effusions. Postgrad Med J. 2004;80(943):262–6.
37. Mayosi BM, Burgess LJ, Doubell AF. Tuberculous pericarditis. Circulation. 2005;112(23):3608–16.
38. Mayosi BM, Ntsekhe M, Bosch J, Pandie S, Jung H, Gumedze F, et al. Prednisolone and Mycobacterium indicus pranii in tuberculous pericarditis. N Engl J Med. 2014;371(12):1121–30.
39. Sagrista-Sauleda J, Permanyer-Miralda G, Soler-Soler J. Tuberculous pericarditis: ten year experience with a prospective

protocol for diagnosis and treatment. J Am Coll Cardiol. 1988; 11(4):724–8.

40. Reuter H, Burgess LJ, Doubell AF. Role of chest radiography in diagnosing patients with tuberculous pericarditis. Cardiovasc J S Afr. 2005;16(2):108–11.

41. Reuter H, Burgess L, van Vuuren W, Doubell A. Diagnosing tuberculous pericarditis. QJM. 2006;99(12):827–39.

42. Trautner BW, Darouiche RO. Tuberculous pericarditis: optimal diagnosis and management. Clin Infect Dis. 2001;33(7):954–61.

43. Tuon FF, Litvoc MN, Lopes MI. Adenosine deaminase and tuberculous pericarditis--a systematic review with meta-analysis. Acta Trop. 2006;99(1):67–74.

44. Rooney JJ, Crocco JA, Lyons HA. Tuberculous pericarditis. Ann Intern Med. 1970;72(1):73–81.

45. Uthaman B, Endrys J, Abushaban L, Khan S, Anim JT. Percutaneous pericardial biopsy: technique, efficacy, safety, and value in the management of pericardial effusion in children and adolescents. Pediatr Cardiol. 1997;18(6):414–8.

46. Quale JM, Lipschik GY, Heurich AE. Management of tuberculous pericarditis. Ann Thorac Surg. 1987;43(6):653–5.

47. Teo HE, Peh WC. Skeletal tuberculosis in children. Pediatr Radiol. 2004;34(11):853–60.

48. Vohra R, Kang HS, Dogra S, Saggar RR, Sharma R. Tuberculous osteomyelitis. J Bone Joint Surg Br. 1997;79(4):562–6.

49. Watts HG, Lifeso RM. Tuberculosis of bones and joints. J Bone Joint Surg Am. 1996;78(2):288–98.

50. Allali F, Mahfoud-Filali S, Hajjaj-Hassouni N. Lymphocytic joint fluid in tuberculous arthritis. A review of 30 cases. Joint Bone Spine. 2005;72(4):319–21.

51. New York City Department of Health and Mental Hygiene Bureau of Tuberculosis Control. Tuberculosis (TB): Clinical Policies & Protocols. 2008. Available at: http://www.nyc.gov/html/doh/html/diseases/tb-hosp-manual.shtml. Accessed 1 Feb 2015.

52. Daher Ede F, da Silva GB, Barros Jr EJ. Renal tuberculosis in the modern era. Am J Trop Med Hyg. 2013;88(1):54–64.

53. Abbara A, Davidson RN. Medscape. Etiology and management of genitourinary tuberculosis. Nat Rev Urol. 2011;8(12):678–88.

54. Hillemann D, Rusch-Gerdes S, Boehme C, Richter E. Rapid molecular detection of extrapulmonary tuberculosis by the automated GeneXpert MTB/RIF system. J Clin Microbiol. 2011;49(4):1202–5.

55. Kapoor VK. Abdominal tuberculosis. Postgrad Med J. 1998; 74(874):459–67.
56. Villalon C, Quezada F, Hartmann J, Roa JC, Urrejola G. Synchronous ileocecal and duodenal tuberculosis: case report and review of the literature. Int J Colorectal Dis. 2014;29(8): 1027–8.
57. Rao YG, Pande GK, Sahni P, Chattopadhyay TK. Gastroduodenal tuberculosis management guidelines, based on a large experience and a review of the literature. Can J Surg. 2004;47(5): 364–8.
58. Poyrazoglu OK, Timurkaan M, Yalniz M, Ataseven H, Dogukan M, Bahcecioglu IH. Clinical review of 23 patients with tuberculous peritonitis: presenting features and diagnosis. J Dig Dis. 2008;9(3):170–4.
59. Manohar A, Simjee AE, Haffejee AA, Pettengell KE. Symptoms and investigative findings in 145 patients with tuberculous peritonitis diagnosed by peritoneoscopy and biopsy over a five year period. Gut. 1990;31(10):1130–2.
60. Kokuto H, Sasaki Y, Yoshimatsu S, Mizuno K, Yi L, Mitarai S. Detection of Mycobacterium tuberculosis (MTB) in fecal specimens from adults diagnosed with pulmonary tuberculosis using the Xpert MTB/rifampicin test. Open Forum Infect Dis. 2015;2(2):ofv074.
61. Marshall JB. Tuberculosis of the gastrointestinal tract and peritoneum. Am J Gastroenterol. 1993;88(7):989–99.
62. Vadwai V, Boehme C, Nabeta P, Shetty A, Alland D, Rodrigues C. Xpert MTB/RIF: a new pillar in diagnosis of extrapulmonary tuberculosis? J Clin Microbiol. 2011;49(7):2540–5.
63. Riquelme A, Calvo M, Salech F, Valderrama S, Pattillo A, Arellano M, et al. Value of adenosine deaminase (ADA) in ascitic fluid for the diagnosis of tuberculous peritonitis: a meta-analysis. J Clin Gastroenterol. 2006;40(8):705–10.
64. Bravo FG, Gotuzzo E. Cutaneous tuberculosis. Clin Dermatol. 2007;25(2):173–80.
65. Santos JB, Figueiredo AR, Ferraz CE, Oliveira MH, Silva PG, Medeiros VL. Cutaneous tuberculosis: epidemiologic, etiopathogenic and clinical aspects - part I. An Bras Dermatol. 2014; 89(2):219–28.
66. Hay RJ. Cutaneous infection with Mycobacterium tuberculosis: how has this altered with the changing epidemiology of tuberculosis? Curr Opin Infect Dis. 2005;18(2):93–5.

67. Dias MF, Bernardes Filho F, Quaresma MV, Nascimento LV, Nery JA, Azulay DR. Update on cutaneous tuberculosis. An Bras Dermatol. 2014;89(6):925–38.
68. Sharma SK, Mohan A, Sharma A, Mitra DK. Miliary tuberculosis: new insights into an old disease. Lancet Infect Dis. 2005; 5(7):415–30.
69. Centers for Disease Control and Prevention. Reported Tuberculosis in the United States. 2013. Available at: http://www. cdc.gov/tb/statistics/. Accessed 1 Feb 2015.
70. Rieder HL, Snider Jr DE, Cauthen GM. Extrapulmonary tuberculosis in the United States. Am Rev Respir Dis. 1990;141(2): 347–51.
71. Mert A, Bilir M, Tabak F, Ozaras R, Ozturk R, Senturk H, et al. Miliary tuberculosis: clinical manifestations, diagnosis and outcome in 38 adults. Respirology. 2001;6(3):217–24.

Chapter 5
Public Health Issues

David W. Dowdy and Jonathan E. Golub

5.1 Introduction

Tuberculosis has been a public health problem for centuries, and with an estimated two billion people living with latent infection, it will continue to wreak havoc in vulnerable populations. Strategies exist that can lessen the burden by treating those with latent infection, detecting and treating active disease earlier, and controlling transmission in congregate settings. Focusing efforts on high-risk populations and settings is likely to impact incidence more than in the general population and is likely more feasible [1]. We briefly review three key public health issues that if properly addressed have the potential to significantly impact the global tuberculosis burden: infection control, contact tracing, and preventive therapy.

D.W. Dowdy (✉)
Department of Epidemiology, Johns Hopkins Bloomberg School of Public Health, 615 N. Wolfe St. Suite E6531, Baltimore, MD 21205, USA
e-mail: ddowdy1@jhmi.edu

J.E. Golub
Medicine/Infectious Disease, Johns Hopkins School of Medicine, 1550 Orleans St. 1M.10, Baltimore, MD 21231, USA
e-mail: jgolub@jhmi.edu

J.H. Grosset, R.E. Chaisson (eds.), *Handbook of Tuberculosis*, 119
DOI 10.1007/978-3-319-26273-4_5,
© Springer International Publishing Switzerland 2017

5.2   Infection Control

The risk of acquiring TB infection and disease, per person-year, is known to be highest in congregate settings, including prisons, mines, and healthcare institutions. A review of active TB in prisons across high-prevalence countries found that case notification rates ranged from 2,400 to 7,000 per 100,000/year, a remarkable 5 % risk of TB disease for every year incarcerated [2]. Similar rates of TB disease (≥3 % per year) were reported in a large cluster-randomized trial of isoniazid preventive therapy in the gold mines of South Africa [3] and in a countrywide investigation of TB in Malawian healthcare workers [4]. Despite these exceptionally high incidence rates of TB disease among populations that are readily accessible to intervention, infection control remains a neglected component of most strategies to end TB.

The link between nosocomial transmission and drug-resistant TB is worthy of specific mention. Since 1990, a number of hospital-related outbreaks of multidrug-resistant (MDR) TB have been reported, often in conjunction with high prevalence of HIV (though a link between HIV and MDR-TB has not been conclusively demonstrated) [5, 6]. Many of these epidemics were effectively controlled following the implementation of strict infection control policies and aggressive campaigns to diagnose and treat MDR-TB. Most recently, concern has been raised about a highly lethal epidemic of extensively drug-resistant (XDR) TB in the South African province of KwaZulu-Natal – an epidemic that also appears to have its roots in nosocomial transmission [7]. Healthcare workers in low-income countries have been estimated to have an occupationally attributable risk of TB infection (not disease) of over 5 % per year [8]. When much of this exposure is to drug-resistant TB, it is understandable why TB exposure is often a major source of low morale among healthcare workers in high-burden settings. Similar to hospitals, prisons have been strongly implicated in the emergence of exceptionally high levels of MDR-TB in the former Soviet Union [9]. The role of congregate settings – especially healthcare and correctional facilities – in catalyzing epidemics of drug-resistant TB is only further motivation to prioritize effective infection control policies.

The principles of TB infection control are well established, particularly for healthcare settings [10]. These include a three-step hierarchy of administrative controls, environmental controls, and respiratory protection [11]. Administrative controls include the development of an infection control plan, assigning responsibility for enacting the plan to a specific individual or individuals, quality assurance, regular training of both patients and staff, screening of those at highest risk for TB infection, decontamination of high-risk equipment, use of infection control data to improve practices, and coordination of efforts between institutional and external (state, provincial, or national) TB control officials. The cornerstone of environmental control is the provision of natural ventilation (with open windows and doors) for all individuals in congregate settings with clinical suspicion of active TB; natural ventilation has been estimated to provide 28 air changes per hour, over twice that of mechanically ventilated negative-pressure rooms [12]. In settings where natural ventilation is impractical and resources are sufficient, additional effective environmental controls include airborne infection isolation (AII) rooms, high-efficiency particulate air (HEPA) filters, and ultraviolet germicidal irradiation (UVGI) [13]. Finally, respiratory protection includes the use of respirators (e.g., N95 masks) with the capacity to filter out particles of very small size, typically at least 0.3 microns, with high efficiency. Importantly, environmental controls and respiratory protection are far less effective in the absence of strong administrative controls as a foundation.

Properly implemented infection control practices are known to be highly effective in preventing the transmission of *M. tuberculosis*. Mathematical models have suggested that infection control practices can reduce the probability of TB infection during high-risk procedures such as autopsy by over 95 % [14]. The use of UVGI alone has been shown to reduce the risk of hospital-transmitted TB infection and disease among guinea pigs by 60–75 % [15]. A widely publicized example of effective infection control occurred at Jackson Memorial Hospital in Miami, Florida, USA [16]. A nosocomial epidemic of MDR-TB at that facility was recognized in May 1990, after which recommended infection control measures were strictly implemented. Although 15 cases had occurred in the preceding 5 months, following implementation of infection control measures in accordance with recommended guidelines, no additional cases of MDR-TB could be traced to ongoing transmission within the hospital (Fig. 5.1). Furthermore, within a year of implementing those measures, the rate of tuberculin skin test (TST) conversions among workers on the HIV ward fell to zero.

In summary, residents of high-risk settings – including prisoners, miners, and hospital patients – are at exceptionally high risk of developing TB, especially drug-resistant forms. Infection control measures – which consist of administrative controls, environmental controls, and respiratory protection – are well described and have been proven to dramatically reduce the risk of TB transmission in such settings. Nevertheless, infection control continues to be deprioritized in national and global plans to fight TB epidemics. Further evaluation of the population-level impact achievable from guideline-based infection control measures in high-prevalence congregate settings should be emphasized [17].

5.3   Contact Tracing

The World Health Organization (WHO) recommended "Three Is" strategy for combating HIV-associated TB includes infection control, isoniazid preventive therapy, and intensified case finding for TB (Fig. 5.2) [18]. Closely linked to intensified case finding (in the case of HIV-associated TB) is systematic screening for TB [19], defined as "the systematic identification of people with suspected active TB, in a predetermined target group, using tests, examinations, or other procedures that can be applied rapidly" [20]. Among risk

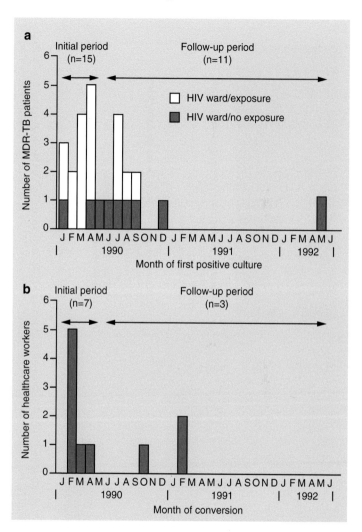

FIG. 5.1 (**a**) Distribution of multidrug-resistant *Mycobacterium tuberculosis* (MDR-TB) patients on HIV ward by date of first positive MDR-TB culture; (**b**) Distribution of healthcare workers with tuberculin skin test conversions (Reproduced with permission from Wenger et al. [16]. ©1995 Elsevier. All rights reserved)

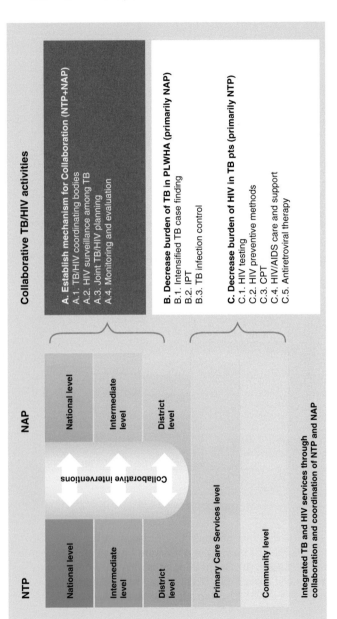

Fig. 5.2 World Health Organization (WHO) strategy for addressing HIV-associated TB. The strategy consists of integration between the National TB Program (NTP) and National AIDS Program (NAP) at all levels, an explicit mechanism for collaboration, specific measures to decrease the burden of TB in people living with HIV/AIDS (PLWHA) - the "three I's" of intensified TB case finding, IPT, and infection control, and efforts to reduce the burden of HIV among patients with TB

groups to be targeted for systematic screening, none carries a stronger evidence base or global recommendation than household and other close contacts of individuals with known active TB.

In low- and middle-income settings, individuals living in the same household as a case of active TB have an esti-mated prevalence of active TB between 2 and 4 % and a prevalence of TB infection of about 50 % [21]. In the first year following exposure, the incidence of active TB ranges from 0.5 % in high-income countries to 1.5 % in low- and middle-income countries – and this risk of active TB remains substantially elevated for at least 5 years (Fig. 5.3). Interestingly, studies in South Africa and Peru have esti-mated that less than half of all household contacts with active TB result from transmission links with the index case [22, 23]. This proportion of linked transmission is substan-tially greater among children and adolescents [24], as well as in low-burden settings [25]. These findings suggest that households containing one case of active TB may serve as markers for high levels of TB transmission in the surround-ing community or social network.

Household contact tracing generally consists of fieldwork-ers visiting the home of an individual diagnosed with active TB and screening all household members for active (and often latent) TB. Alternatively, household members may be asked to return to a clinic to be screened. Upon ruling out active TB, provision of preventive therapy is generally recommended for household members with evidence of TB infection (e.g., a positive tuberculin skin test), those who are infected with HIV, and children under the age of 5 [26]. Despite strong recommendations to perform household con-tact tracing, global implementation of this strategy in high-burden settings remains poor. Concerns about cost are one major reason for this slow scale-up of a proven intervention; although modeling analyses have suggested that screening childhood contacts is likely to be highly cost-effective even in high-burden settings [27], data on the cost-effectiveness of contact investigation in practice remains sparse.

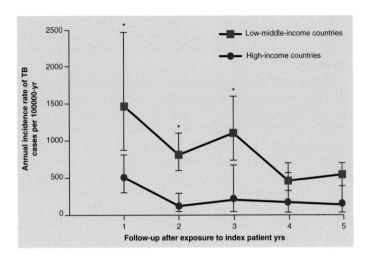

FIG. 5.3 Annual incidence rate of tuberculosis (TB) in contacts by year of follow-up, according to country income. World Bank Income Gross National Income per capita: low income ($\leq$\$1,005 per yr); lower-middle income (\$1,006 to \$3,975 per yr); upper-middle income (\$3,976 to \$12,275 per yr); high income ($\geq$\$12,276 per yr). *: $p < 0.05$, statistically significant difference between contacts from high compared to low- and middle-income countries (Reproduced with permission from Fox et al. [21]. ©European Respiratory Journal)

When performing household contact investigations, one important consideration is that household contacts with active TB often have earlier forms of the disease, with different clinical manifestations. For example, in one evaluation of contact tracing in South Africa, only 6 % of active TB among household contacts was sputum smear positive, and the majority of culture-confirmed TB occurred in asymptomatic individuals [28]. Since symptom screening appears to carry very poor sensitivity in the setting of contact tracing and performance of universal culture among all household contacts is unlikely to be feasible, evaluation of algorithms that make use of sensitive screening tests (e.g., chest X-ray) is an important priority.

Household contact tracing plus effective treatment for contacts detected with TB disease or infection has the potential to reduce TB burden at the population level, though this effect has not been conclusively demonstrated with empirical data. Perhaps the largest evaluation to date of a household-centered intervention as a means to reduce TB incidence was the Zambia/South Africa TB and AIDS Reduction (ZAMSTAR) study, a cluster-randomized trial of 24 communities containing nearly one million individuals [29]. In this study, household-based TB and HIV care reduced the prevalence of TB disease by 18 % and the incidence of TB infection among schoolchildren by 55 % over 4 years, though these differences were not statistically significant. Similar results (a statistically significant 15 % decline in TB incidence over 5 years) were seen in a smaller randomized trial of enhanced household screening and preventive therapy in Rio de Janeiro, Brazil [30]. A subsequent mathematical model estimated that a household contact tracing campaign could reduce TB incidence at the population level by 2–3 % per year for 5 years or more and that this impact could be doubled by the use of preventive therapy in those found not to have active TB [31]. Thus, while contact tracing may be an efficient, effective, and cost-effective intervention, it is unlikely on its own to reverse TB epidemics at the community level. Household contact tracing should therefore be seen as part of a comprehensive strategy that also includes infection control, preventive therapy, improved diagnosis and treatment, and the use of data to target TB control resources appropriately.

A question of emerging interest is whether household contacts of people with MDR-TB are at increased risk of transmission relative to contacts of drug-susceptible cases. Early studies suggested that the risk of TB infection and disease among contacts of MDR-TB cases was similar to that among contacts of cases with drug-susceptible TB, despite longer duration of contact to MDR-TB cases [32]. More recently, a prospective cohort study of over 3,400 household contacts in Peru suggested that contacts of MDR-TB cases had only half the hazard of TB disease as contacts of drug-susceptible TB cases [33]. These and similar emerging results will be useful in helping to assess the relative transmissibility of MDR-TB, as well as the value of contact investigation strategies that focus specifically on people exposed to MDR-TB cases.

Ultimately, if we are to develop effective strategies to end TB epidemics, we must first start with those individuals at highest risk of having or developing active TB. Household contacts of people diagnosed with TB are one such high-risk group, and screening these individuals for active TB is not only universally recommended but also universally seen as a cornerstone of TB elimination strategies in high-income settings. Household contact tracing is an effective and likely cost-effective method for identifying individuals with active TB before they become ill and highly infectious, and our best available evidence suggests that this strategy likely has meaningful population-level impact as well. Finding ways to integrate household contact tracing into routine TB activities in high-burden settings must therefore be seen as a critical step to developing comprehensive local strategies capable of rapidly bending the TB epidemic curve.

5.4   Preventive Therapy

Potentially the most impactful strategy for tuberculosis control is to prevent TB from developing in the estimated one-quarter of the world who are latently infected [34]. However, identifying those at greatest risk of reactivation from a biomarker perspective remains elusive. From an epidemiologic perspective, we have some clues, the strongest of which is that HIV-infected patients are at great risk of developing TB if untreated. Treatment with antiretroviral therapy (ART) has proven to reduce TB risk markedly, across CD4 strata [35], but risk still remains high among patients receiving ART.

Treatment of latent tuberculosis infection with isoniazid (INH) or other antituberculosis medications reduces the risk of subsequent tuberculosis by 60–90 % [36]. Provision of treatment for latent infection to people at high risk of developing tuberculosis is an important adjunct to case identification and treatment in reducing tuberculosis incidence in a community and has been used extensively in the USA and Europe. In the USA, INH preventive therapy is targeted at close contacts of infectious cases, individuals with HIV and latent tuberculosis infection, recent tuberculin converters, and other tuberculin-positive people at high risk of developing active tuberculosis [37]. For the past two decades, recommendations in the USA have stated that 9 months of daily INH is the most effective duration (CDC), based primarily on Comstock's analysis of INH clinical trial outcomes [38]. Adherence to a 9-month regimen is challenging; thus, shorter courses of therapy are desired. A recent study conducted in several low to moderate TB incident countries reported that a 3-month once-weekly combination of rifapentine and isoniazid was not inferior to the standard 9-month INH regimen [39]. The 3-month regimen also had a higher adherence rate, was more cost-effective [40], and was less hepatotoxic [41] compared to the 9-month INH regimen. Most recently, results from the same study have shown that the 3-month regimen also protects HIV-infected patients [42].

In low- and middle-income countries (LMICs), the use of treatment for latent infection is very limited and, if used at all, is usually directed only at young children living in households with smear-positive cases. The HIV epidemic has changed the dynamics of tuberculosis in many LMICs, and evidence now suggests that provision of INH to HIV-infected patients receiving HAART can significantly reduce TB risk [43–46]. Effective control of tuberculosis in HIV-endemic areas requires treatment of latent infection if true control is to be achieved [47, 48], though the durability of preventive therapy for HIV-infected patients is variable and at least partially dependent upon the TB incidence and the corresponding likelihood of reinfection in the area. Durability of IPT in the pre-HIV era was shown clearly in early trials in Alaska where annual infection rates and TB incidence rival present day South Africa, and protection from TB disease remained for 20 years [49]. However, the impact of HIV on progression of TB infection, along with recent trial results, suggests that lifetime preventive therapy may be required for HIV-infected patients living in high TB incident areas. In a trial in Botswana, HIV-infected patients randomized to receive IPT for 3 years had a 56 % reduction in TB risk, though the protection conferred was limited to TST-positive participants [50]. A follow-up study revealed that the benefit of 3 years of IPT declined significantly posttrial. A trial in South Africa, which included only TST-positive patients, reported no benefit of long-term IPT in the intent-to-treat analysis, but an as-treated analysis reported 58 % protection among patients who were actively receiving long-term IPT compared with those who only receive 6 months of IPT [51]. An Indian trial found no benefit of long-term IPT compared to a 6-month regimen of isoniazid and ethambutol [52]. India has considerably lower incidence and prevalence of TB which may have impacted risk of reinfection. A follow-up analysis of the THRio study in Brazil, where TB incidence is lower than India and one-tenth of what is seen in South Africa, has shown that a 6-month regimen of IPT can significantly curtail TB risk among HIV-infected patients [53].

Despite strong evidence that preventive therapy for tuberculosis can be markedly beneficial to HIV-infected patients, many implementation barriers have limited uptake. WHO reports that globally in 2014, just under 1 million people living with HIV received IPT, and two-thirds of those were in South Africa [54] (Fig. 5.4). These barriers include challenges in ruling out active tuberculosis disease prior to initiation of IPT, fear of developing drug resistance, and concerns of serious side effects such as hepatotoxicity [55, 56] (Table 5.1). However, evidence suggests that drug-resistant disease is rarely detected [57], and side effects have been consistently minimal [58] even in studies of long-term IPT use [50, 52, 56]. Many preventive therapy guidelines in high-incidence settings include the tuberculin skin test as a tool to determine who should initiate therapy. The TST has been an operational barrier for decades [59], as it requires trained

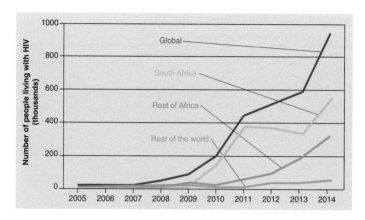

personnel to administer and read a return visit by the patient and cold chain maintenance [55]. Most damning is the low sensitivity of TST, particularly in HIV-infected patients, thus limiting confidence in the test as a determination for IPT initiation. In the most recent WHO guidelines for IPT, WHO recommends IPT for all HIV-infected patients in high-burden countries irrespective of TST status [60]. However, in recognition of studies showing that TST-positive patients do benefit most from IPT [50, 61], TST is recommended if a current program is in place.

Preventive therapy has remained a low priority in almost all settings, but particularly in LMICs where detecting and treating active disease is the number one objective, leaving few resources for preventive therapy. Although better diagnostics for detecting latent infection, discovery of biomarkers that predict who will develop active disease, and effective short-course regimens will all significantly improve implementation of preventive therapy, current tools, and strategies and, if better implemented, can have a huge impact on the TB epidemic in all settings.

TABLE 5.1 Barriers to implementation of tuberculosis preventive therapy and proposed responses

	Proposed responses
Clinical	
Excluding active tuberculosis, especially in HIV-positive patients	The use of clinical algorithms, more use of chest X-rays
Need for tuberculin or other testing [IGRA (interferon γ release assay)]	Develop new simple tests that are more predictive of subsequent active tuberculosis, improve worldwide production of tuberculin, treat high-risk patients without testing
Poor adherence and completion of preventive therapy	The use of short-course regimens and supervision of therapy
Drug toxicity	Encourage monthly monitoring and patient education
Perceived risk of acquiring drug resistance	Available evidence suggests that this is not a problem
Health system	
The absence of consistent guidelines	Harmonized worldwide and national guidelines Development of preventive therapy instruments
Inadequately trained staff	Enhanced training for doctors, nurses, and other health workers
Stock-outs of drugs and diagnostics (tuberculin skin test or IGRA)	Strengthened supply chain
Poor surveillance and reporting	Better health information systems, increased monitoring and assessment

Table 5.1 (continued)

	Proposed responses
Inadequate funding	Expansion of vertical health programs to address tuberculosis prevention (e.g., HIV prevention of mother-to-child transmission), with benchmarks for disease control; more integration of tuberculosis control into primary health care
Policy and advocacy	
The absence of priority for prevention, with emphasis on proportion of active cases treated	Realignment of tuberculosis control programs to incorporate prevention, with performance assessment linked to incidence
Inadequate investment in basic, clinical and implementation research and training	Increased funding for research
The absence of advocacy and demand from groups most at risk	Education and empowerment of at-risk group, including people with HIV and families

5.5 Conclusion

Novel public health strategies are needed if the global tuberculosis burden is going to decline to the levels outlined in the WHO End TB Strategy over the next two decades. The current rate of decline suggests that these goals may be difficult to reach. However, many strategies have been successful at reducing TB burden in distinct populations and if properly operationalized and scaled can have greater impact. Controlling tuberculosis transmission in congregate settings and hospitals, searching for and treating household contacts of TB cases for both latent and active TB, and providing preventive therapy to at-risk populations can each, and cumulatively together, markedly impact the global epidemic. New strategies, tools, and drugs remain top priorities, but implementing those that we already have at our disposal must be considered a necessity in all settings.

References

1. Dowdy DW, Golub JE, Chaisson RE, Saraceni V. Heterogeneity in tuberculosis transmission and the role of geographic hotspots in propagating epidemics. Proc Natl Acad USA. 2012;109(24): 9557–62.
2. Coninx R, Maher D, Reyes H, Grzemska M. Tuberculosis in prisons in countries with high prevalence. BMJ. 2000;320(7232): 440–2.
3. Churchyard GJ, Fielding KL, Lewis JJ, Coetzee L, Corbett EL, Godfrey-Faussett P, Hayes RJ, Chaisson RE, Grant AD, Thibela TB Study Team. A trial of mass isoniazid preventive therapy for tuberculosis control. N Engl J Med. 2014;370(4):301–10.
4. Harries AD, Nyirenda TE, Banerjee A, Boeree MJ, Salaniponi FM. Tuberculosis in health care workers in Malawi. Trans R Soc Trop Med Hyg. 1999;93(1):32–5.
5. Centers for Disease Control (CDC). Nosocomial transmission of multidrug-resistant tuberculosis among HIV-infected persons – Florida and New York, 1988–1991. MMWR Morb Mortal Wkly Rep. 1991;40(34):585–91.
6. Ritacco V, Di Lonardo M, Reniero A, Ambroggi M, Barrera L, Dambrosi A, Lopez B, Isola N, de Kantor IN. Nosocomial spread of human immunodeficiency virus-related multidrug-resistant tuberculosis in Buenos Aires. J Infect Dis. 1997;176(3): 637–42.
7. Gandhi NR, Moll A, Sturm AW, Pawinski R, Govender T, Lalloo U, Zeller K, Andrews J, Friedland G. Extensively drug-resistant tuberculosis as a cause of death in patients co-infected with tuberculosis and HIV in a rural area of South Africa. Lancet. 2006;368(9547):1575–80.

8. Menzies D, Joshi R, Pai M. Risk of tuberculosis infection and disease associated with work in health care settings. Int J Tuberc Lung Dis. 2007;11(6):593–605.

9. Portaels F, Rigouts L, Bastian I. Addressing multidrug-resistant tuberculosis in penitentiary hospitals and in the general population of the former Soviet Union. Int J Tuberc Lung Dis. 1999;3(7): 582–8.

10. Jensen PA, Lambert LA, Iademarco MF, Ridzon R; CDC. Guidelines for preventing the transmission of Mycobacterium tuberculosis in health-care settings, 2005. MMWR Recomm Rep. 2005; 54(RR-17):1–141.

11. Bock NN, Jensen PA, Miller B, Nardell E. Tuberculosis infection control in resource-limited settings in the era of expanding HIV care and treatment. J Infect Dis. 2007;196 Suppl 1:S108–13.

12. Escombe AR, Oeser CC, Gilman RH, Navincopa M, Ticona E, Pan W, Martínez C, Chacaltana J, Rodríguez R, Moore DA, Friedland JS, Evans CA. Natural ventilation for the prevention of airborne contagion. PLoS Med. 2007;4(2), e68.

13. Kowalski W. Ultraviolet germicidal irradiation handbook. Heidelberg: Springer, 2009. Gammaitoni L, Nucci MC. Using a mathematical model to evaluate the efficacy of TB control measures. Emerg Infect Dis. 1997;3(3):335–42.

14. Gammaitoni L, Nucci MC. Using a mathematical model to evaluate the efficacy of TB control measures. Emerg Infect Dis. 1997;3(3):335–42.

15. Escombe AR, Moore DA, Gilman RH, Navincopa M, Ticona E, Mitchell B, Noakes C, Martínez C, Sheen P, Ramirez R, Quino W, Gonzalez A, Friedland JS, Evans CA. Upper-room ultraviolet light and negative air ionization to prevent tuberculosis transmission. PLoS Med. 2009;6(3), e43.

16. Wenger PN, Otten J, Breeden A, Orfas D, Beck-Sague CM, Jarvis WR. Control of nosocomial transmission of multidrug-resistant Mycobacterium tuberculosis among healthcare workers and HIV-infected patients. Lancet. 1995;345(8944):235–40.

17. Basu S, Andrews JR, Poolman EM, et al. Prevention of nosocomial transmission of extensively drug-resistant tuberculosis in rural South African district hospitals: an epidemiological modelling study. Lancet. 2007;370(9597):1500–7.

18. Three I's Meeting WHO. Report of a joint World Health Organization HIV/AIDS and TB Department Meeting. 2–4 April, Geneva, Switzerland. Geneva: WHO; 2008.

19. Kranzer K, Afnan-Holmes H, Tomlin K, et al. The benefits to communities and individuals of screening for active tuberculosis

disease: a systematic review. Int J Tuberc Lung Dis. 2013;17(4): 432–46.

20. World Health Organization. Systematic screening for active tuberculosis: principles and recommendations. Geneva: WHO; 2013.

21. Fox GJ, Barry SE, Britton WJ, Marks GB. Contact investigation for tuberculosis: a systematic review and meta-analysis. Eur Respir J. 2013;41(1):140–56.

22. Verver S, Warren RM, Munch Z, et al. Proportion of tuberculosis transmission that takes place in households in a high-incidence area. Lancet. 2004;363(9404):212–4.

23. Brooks-Pollock E, Becerra MC, Goldstein E, Cohen T, Murray MB. Epidemiologic inference from the distribution of tuberculosis cases in households in Lima. Peru J Infect Dis. 2011;203(11): 1582–9.

24. Zelner JL, Murray MB, Becerra MC, et al. Age-specific risks of tuberculosis infection from household and community exposures and opportunities for interventions in a high-burden setting. Am J Epidemiol. 2014;180(8):853–61.

25. Behr MA, Hopewell PC, Paz EA, Kawamura LM, Schecter GF, Small PM. Predictive value of contact investigation for identifying recent transmission of Mycobacterium tuberculosis. Am J Respir Crit Care Med. 1998;158(2):465–9.

26. World Health Organization. Recommendations for investigating contacts of persons with infectious tuberculosis in low- and middle-income countries. Geneva: WHO; 2012.

27. Mandalakas AM, Hesseling AC, Gie RP, Schaaf HS, Marais BJ, Sinanovic E. Modelling the cost-effectiveness of strategies to prevent tuberculosis in child contacts in a high-burden setting. Thorax. 2013;68(3):247–55.

28. Shapiro AE, Variava E, Rakgokong MH, et al. Community-based targeted case finding for tuberculosis and HIV in household contacts of patients with tuberculosis in South Africa. Am J Respir Crit Care Med. 2012;185(10):1110–6.

29. Ayles H, Muyoyeta M, Du Toit E, et al. Effect of household and community interventions on the burden of tuberculosis in southern Africa: the ZAMSTAR community-randomised trial. Lancet. 2013;382(9899):1183–94.

30. Cavalcante SC, Durovni B, Barnes GL, et al. Community-randomized trial of enhanced DOTS for tuberculosis control in Rio de Janeiro. Brazil Int J Tuberc Lung Dis. 2010;14(2):203–9.

31. Kasaie P, Andrews JR, Kelton WD, Dowdy DW. Timing of tuberculosis transmission and the impact of household contact tracing. An agent-based simulation model. Am J Respir Crit Care Med. 2014;189(7):845–52.

32. Teixeira L, Perkins MD, Johnson JL, et al. Infection and disease among household contacts of patients with multidrug-resistant tuberculosis. Int J Tuberc Lung Dis. 2001;5(4):321–8.

33. Grandjean L, Gilman RH, Martin L, et al. Transmission of Multidrug-Resistant and Drug-Susceptible Tuberculosis within Households: A Prospective Cohort Study. PLoS Med. 2015;12(6), e1001843.

34. Houben RMGJ, Dodd PJ. The Global Burden of Latent Tuberculosis Infection: A Re-estimation Using Mathematical Modelling. PLOS Medicine. 2016.

35. Suthar AB, Lawn SD, del Amo J, et al. Antiretroviral therapy for prevention of tuberculosis in adults with HIV: a systematic review and meta-analysis. PLoS Med. 2012;9(7), e1001270.

36. Ferebee S. Controlled chemoprophylaxis trials in tuberculosis: a general review. Adv Tuberc Res. 1970;17:28–106.

37. ATS/CDC. Targeted tuberculin testing and treatment of latent tuberculosis in latent tuberculosis infection. MMWR. 2000; 49(RR06):1–54.

38. Comstock GW. How much isoniazid is needed for prevention of tuberculosis among immuncompetent adults? Int J Tuberc Lung Dis. 1999;3(10):847–50.

39. Sterling TR, Villarino ME, Borisov AS, et al. Three months of rifapentine and isoniazid for latent tuberculosis infection. N Engl J Med. 2011;365:2155–66.

40. Shepardson D, Marks SM, Chesson H, et al. Cost-effectiveness of a 12-dose regimen for treating latent tuberculosis infection in the United States. Int J Tuberc Lung Dis. 2013;17(12):1531–7.

41. Bliven-Sizemore EE, Sterling TR, Sang N, et al. Three months of weekly rifapentine plus isoniazid is less hepatotoxic than nine months of daily isoniazid for LTBI. Int J Tuberc Lung Dis. 1999;2015:1039–44.

42. Sterling TR, Scott NA, Miro JM, et al. Tuberculosis Trials Consortium, the AIDS Clinical Trials Group for the PREVENT TB Trial (TBTC Study 26ACTG 5259). Three months of weekly rifapentine and isoniazid for treatment of Mycobacterium tuberculosis infection in HIV-coinfected persons. AIDS. 2016;30(10):1607–15.

43. Golub JE, Saraceni V, Cavalcante SC, et al. The impact of antiretroviral therapy and isoniazid preventive therapy on tubercu-

138   D.W. Dowdy and J.E. Golub

losis incidence in HIV-infected patients in Rio de Janeiro, Brazil. AIDS. 2007;21:1441–8.

44. Golub JE, Pronyk P, Mohapi L, et al. Isoniazid preventive therapy, HAART and tuberculosis risk in HIV-infected adults in South Africa: a prospective cohort. AIDS. 2009;23(5): 631–6.

45. Rangaka MX, Wilkinson RJ, Boulle A, et al. Isoniazid plus antiretroviral therapy to prevent tuberculosis: a randomised double-blind, placebo-controlled trial. Lancet. 2014;384:682–90.

46. Temprano ANRS. 12136 Study Group. A trial of early antiretrovirals and isoniazid preventive therapy in Africa. N Engl J Med. 2015;373:808–22.

47. Dye C, Glaziou P, Floyd K, Raviglione M. Prospects for tuberculosis elimination. Annu Rev Public Health. 2013;34:271–86.

48. Dowdy DW, Golub JE, Saraceni V, et al. Impact of isoniazid preventive therapy for HIV-infected adults in Rio de Janeiro, Brazil: an epidemiological model. J Acquir Immune Defic Syndr. 2014;66(5):552–8.

49. Comstock GW, Baum C, Snider Jr DE. Isoniazid prophylaxis among Alaskan Eskimos: a final report of the bethel isoniazid studies. Am Rev Respir Dis. 1979;119:827–30.

50. Samandari T, Agizew TB, Nyirenda S, et al. 6-month versus 36-month isoniazid preventive treatment for tuberculosis in adults with HIV infection in Botswana: a randomised, double-blind, placebo controlled trial. Lancet. 2011;377:1588–98.

51. Martinson NA, Barnes GL, Moulton LH, et al. New regimens to prevent tuberculosis in adults with HIV infection. N Engl J Med. 2011;365:11–20.

52. Swaminathan S, Menon PA, Gopalan N, et al. Efficacy of a six-month versus a 36-month regimen for prevention of tuberculosis in HIV-infected persons in India: a randomized clinical trial. PLoS One. 2012;7(12), e47400.

53. Golub JE, Cohn S, Saraceni V, et al. Long-term protection from isoniazid preventive therapy for tuberculosis in HIV-infected patients in a medium-burden tuberculosis setting: the TB/HIV in Rio (THRio) study. Clin Infect Dis. 2015;60:639–45.

54. World Health Organization. Global tuberculosis report 2015. 20th ed. WHO/HTM/TB/2015.22.

55. Akolo C, Bada F, Okpokoro E, et al. Debunking the myths perpetuating low implementation of isoniazid preventive therapy amongst human immunodeficiency virus-infected persons. World J Virol. 2015;4(2):105–12.

56. Rangaka M, Cavalcante SC, Marais BJ, et al. Controlling the seedbeds of tuberculosis: diagnosis and treatment of tuberculosis infection. Lancet. 2015;386(10010):2344–53.

57. Balcells ME, Thomas SL, Godfrey-Faussett P, Grant AD. Isoniazid preventive therapy and risk for resistant tuberculosis. Emerg Infect Dis. 2006;12:744–51.

58. Durovni B, Saraceni V, Moulton LH, et al. Effect of improved tuberculosis screening and isoniazid preventive therapy on incidence of tuberculosis and death in patients with HIV in clinics in Rio de Janeiro, Brazil: a stepped wedge, cluster-randomized trial. Lancet Infect Dis. 2013;13(10):852–8.

59. Getahun H, Granich R, Sculier D, et al. Implementation of isoniazid preventive therapy for people living with HIV worldwide: barriers and solutions. AIDS. 2010;24 Suppl 5:S57–65.

60. World Health Organization (WHO) Guidelines for intensified case finding and isoniazid preventive therapy for people living with HIV in resource constrained settings. Geneva. 2011. Available from: http://whqlibdoc.who.int/publications/2011/9789241500708_ eng.pdf.

61. Akolo C, Adetifa I, Shepperd S, Volmink J. Treatment of latent tuberculosis infection in HIV infected persons. Cochrane Database Syst Rev. 2010;1, CD000171.

Chapter 6
Management of Tuberculosis in Special Populations

Nicole Salazar-Austin, Sanjay Jain, and Kelly E. Dooley

6.1 Tuberculosis in HIV-Infected Persons

6.1.1 Epidemiology

Tuberculosis (TB) is the leading cause of death among people living with HIV and/or AIDS (PLWHA) globally [1]. In 2014, of 9.6 million people with incident cases of TB worldwide, 1.2 million (12 %) were HIV infected. And of the 1.5 million TB-related deaths, 400,000 (33 %) had HIV coinfection [2]. Clearly, PLWHA bear a disproportionate burden of TB disease. Unlike other opportunistic infections in which the risk of disease is generally not elevated among those individuals with HIV infection with high CD4 counts, TB incidence increases substantially even within the first year of HIV infection, when CD4 counts are generally high [3]. Risk rises further with progressive immunodeficiency [4]. The

N. Salazar-Austin (✉) • S. Jain • K. E. Dooley (✉)
Pediatric Infectious Diseases and Center for Tuberculosis Research, Johns Hopkins University School of Medicine and Bloomberg School of Public Health, Baltimore, USA
e-mail: sjain5@jhmi.edu; kdooley1@jhmi.edu

J.H. Grosset, R.E. Chaisson (eds.), *Handbook of Tuberculosis*,   141
DOI 10.1007/978-3-319-26273-4_6,
© Springer International Publishing Switzerland 2017

annual risk of development of TB disease among persons
with latent TB infection (LTBI) and untreated HIV infection
is approximately 10 % [5].

6.1.2   Prevention of Tuberculosis Disease

The annual risk of TB disease is 5–10 times higher in persons
with HIV infection than the general population; among individuals with LTBI, HIV is the strongest known risk factor for
progressing to TB disease [6]. However, risk is reduced substantially with treatment of either HIV or LTBI or both [7–
11]. Clearly, provision of antiretroviral therapy (ART) and/or
TB prophylaxis is appropriate to reduce risk of disease in this
population.

Treatment of HIV Infection

In all settings, ART should be provided to all HIV-infected
persons, regardless of CD4 count, insomuch as resources
allow. In high TB burden settings, even among patients with
CD4 counts >350 cells/mm^3, early ART reduces TB incidence
substantially. ART reduces risk of TB in low- and moderate-
burden settings as well [12, 13].

Diagnosis of Latent TB Infection (LTBI)

All persons with HIV infection should be screened for LTBI
at the time of HIV diagnosis and yearly thereafter, given the
high annual risk of TB disease in HIV-infected persons.
Screening can be undertaken using tuberculin skin test (TST)
or with interferon-gamma release assays (IGRAs). While
IGRA may have modestly higher sensitivity than TST among
PLWHA and has higher specificity among persons previously
vaccinated with BCG, serial testing with IGRA presents challenges in this population because spontaneous variability in
test results is common with these tests and may be hard to
interpret [14]. In contrast, with serial TST, a new positive test

may represent either incident infection or pre-existing infection that can now be diagnosed by TST because of enhanced immunologic response to tuberculin resulting from effective HIV treatment. In either case, a new positive TST merits LTBI treatment. Thus, for serial testing for LTBI, in our view, TST is preferable to IGRA. In addition, it should be noted that while there is strong, consistent evidence that isoniazid preventive therapy (IPT) reduces risk of progression to TB disease among persons with TST skin test positivity, no such evidence exists for persons with IGRA test positivity. Overall, the tests have equally poor predictive accuracy for identifying individuals who will (or will not) eventually develop TB disease [15].

TB Prophylactic Therapy

Whom to treat. In high-burden settings, TB prophylactic therapy may provide benefit to individuals with HIV infection, regardless of TST status. While evidence for the benefit of IPT among TST-positive individuals is clear [10, 16], evidence for benefit of IPT among TST-negative individuals in this setting is mixed. While overall, IPT does not appear to provide benefit to PLWHA with negative TST, TST positivity varies by CD4 count, and the test has lower sensitivity in persons with low CD4 counts. In one large meta-analysis of TST responses in PLWHA from multiple continents, TST positivity was as follows: 12 % for CD4 <200, 28 % for CD4 200–499, and 37 % for CD4 ≥ 500 cells/mm³ [17]. This suggests that many persons with advanced HIV/AIDS in high TB incidence areas have LTBI but cannot be diagnosed with TST; these persons are at high risk of progression to active disease and may benefit from prophylaxis [18]. In low- to medium-incidence settings, the benefit of IPT among PLWHA with negative TST results has not been demonstrated. Thus, TB prophylaxis should be offered to all persons with positive TST and may be considered for those individuals with negative TST that live in high-incidence settings and have advanced AIDS. TB prophylaxis should also be offered to close contacts of TB patients, regardless of TST status. Of course TB prophylaxis should only be offered once active disease has been ruled out by symptom screening, chest radiograph, and, when appropriate, sputum testing.

Treatment options. IPT, with isoniazid given at a dose of 5 mg/kg (maximum 300 mg) daily for 9 months, has proven efficacy and is generally well tolerated. In PLWHA, baseline liver function testing is advised [19], and vitamin B6 (pyridoxine) supplementation at a dose of 25–50 mg per day should be provided. Longer treatment for up to 36 months has shown benefit in some high-incidence settings but not others [20, 21]. HIV infection does not appear to increase risk of clinically significant liver toxicity [22]. Other recommended treatment options include once-weekly rifapentine plus isoniazid given for 3 months (rifapentine 900 mg and isoniazid 900 mg once weekly for 12 total doses) [23], 3–4 months of daily isoniazid plus rifampin (isoniazid 5 mg/kg, 300 mg maximum, and rifampin 10 mg/kg, 600 mg maximum), or 4 months of rifampin alone (10 mg/kg, 600 mg maximum) [19, 24]. Both rifampin and rifapentine are strong inducers of metabolizing enzymes, so drug interactions involving these agents are common. Both drugs are safe to use with nucleoside (or nucleotide) reverse transcriptase inhibitors (NRTI) and efavirenz [25, 26]. Rifapentine cannot be used together with protease inhibitors, but rifapentine can be safely coadministered with raltegravir [27]. For details about drug interactions involving rifampin, please see Sect. 6.1.5.

6.1.3   Clinical Presentation of Tuberculosis Disease

Among individuals without significant immunodeficiency, TB manifests in similar fashion to HIV-uninfected individuals, chiefly with pulmonary TB and associated fever, night sweats, weight loss, and productive cough. Extrapulmonary diseases such as pleural effusion, meningitis, lymphadenitis, and pericardial disease are common among HIV-coinfected persons, at all CD4 counts, occurring in 70 % of persons with CD4 count ≤100 and about 30 % of people with CD4 count >300 cells/mm^3 [28, 29]. With advancing immunodeficiency, cavitary disease is less often seen, while disseminated disease, manifest by miliary lung infiltrates and bacteremia with sepsis, is common [28]. In addition, with HIV treatment, previously undiagnosed TB can be "unmasked" as patients recover immunologic function and mount a brisk inflammatory response to *Mycobacterium tuberculosis* bacilli, developing so-called immune reconstitution inflammatory syndrome or IRIS [30]. ART can typically be continued with the addition of anti-TB treatment and steroids (see Sect. 6.1.5).

6.1.4 Diagnosis

As with HIV-uninfected individuals with suspected TB, diagnostic testing is focused on the relevant anatomic site, as directed by symptoms and physical examination findings. If active TB is suspected, a chest radiograph should be performed, even if there are not clear pulmonary manifestations, as concurrent lung disease is common among patients with extrapulmonary disease. Sputum should be collected for smear and culture if there are pulmonary symptoms or suggestive abnormalities on chest imaging. Though patients with advanced immunodeficiency may be less likely to have cavitary lung disease and are, thus, less likely to have sputum that is smear positive for acid-fast bacilli (AFB), culture is still quite sensitive and should be performed. Genotypic tests such as Xpert MTB/RIF have excellent sensitivity for detecting *M. tuberculosis* in the cerebrospinal fluid or lymph node tissue [31], offering another diagnostic option for HIV-infected patients with suspected extrapulmonary disease. In individuals with advanced HIV, lateral flow urine TB lipoarabinomannan (LAM) assays may be helpful for diagnosing disseminated TB [32, 33], but further validation of this test is still required.

6.1.5   Treatment Considerations

Treatment of HIV-related TB

The treatment of drug-sensitive and drug-resistant TB is the same for patients with and without HIV coinfection and is described in detail in previous chapters and in Sect. 6.3, respectively. In brief, for drug-sensitive TB, isoniazid, rifampin, pyrazinamide, and ethambutol (HRZE) are given for 2 months (intensive phase); then, isoniazid and rifampin are given for 4 months (continuation phase). There is evidence that HIV infection is a risk factor for development of acquired resistance, particularly among patients with isoniazid-resistant TB, untreated HIV, and/or intermittent treatment regimens [34, 35]. Thus, for patients with HIV/TB coinfection, TB treatment should be delivered 5–7 days per week, not twice or thrice weekly.

Timing of Initiation of ART

Patients with untreated HIV infection have a significantly higher risk of relapse with standard duration TB treatment than PLWHA on ART or HIV-uninfected persons [36]. Similarly, mortality is higher among patients waiting to start ART until TB treatment is complete compared to those who are treated for HIV and TB concurrently, especially among persons with low CD4 counts [37]. For patients with CD4 counts <50 cells/mm^3, HIV treatment should be initiated within 2 weeks of starting TB therapy, as this improves survival and reduces incidence of new AIDS-defining illnesses compared to starting ART after completion of the intensive phase (8 weeks) of TB therapy [38–40]. Whether or not it is safe or advisable to delay initiation of ART among those patients with CD4 counts above 220 cells/mm^3 is unclear [37, 41]. However, given the overall health benefits of ART for persons of all CD4 counts [42], it is advisable to start it as soon as feasible after initiating TB treatment (within 8–12 weeks), taking into account the challenges of overlapping toxicities, pill burden, coordination of care, and drug interactions.

TB and HIV Regimen Selection

Rifampin, the key sterilizing drug in the regimen for drug-sensitive TB, is a potent inducer of metabolizing enzymes, so its use can result in clinically important drug interactions with companion drugs [43]. In most instances, it is best to use standard TB treatment (HRZE) along with compatible ART regimens, such as two NRTIs plus one of the following: efavirenz (at the standard 600 mg dose) [25], raltegravir (at an increased dose of 800 mg twice daily) [44], or dolutegravir (at an increased dose of 50 mg twice daily) [45]. Alternatively, rifabutin can be used in place of rifampin, and an ART regimen consisting of two NRTIs plus a ritonavir-boosted protease inhibitor can be given; in this case, rifabutin should be given at a reduced dose of 150 mg once daily (rather than a dose of 300 mg daily) because ritonavir inhibits its metabolism [46, 47]. With HIV/TB co-treatment, special attention should be given to potential overlapping toxicities, chief among them hepatotoxicity (rifampin, pyrazinamide, isoniazid, protease inhibitors), central nervous system toxicities (isoniazid, efavirenz), gastrointestinal upset (rifampin, isoniazid, pyrazinamide, protease inhibitors), rash (rifampin, efavirenz), cytopenias (rifabutin, rifampin, zidovudine), and peripheral neuropathy (isoniazid, some NRTI). It is extremely important that coordination of HIV and TB care be undertaken, especially if doses of either TB or HIV drugs are adjusted to mitigate drug interactions [48].

Treatment Response

When patients with HIV-associated TB are treated with standard TB drugs and ART, outcomes are generally similar to those seen among HIV-uninfected persons. However, risk of relapse may be modestly higher [36], even among patients on ART. Some recommend treating for 9 months instead of 6, particularly in patients that have not converted their sputum culture to negative by 2 months of treatment. The population most likely to benefit from prolonged treatment remains ill-defined.

Immune Reconstitution Inflammatory Syndrome (IRIS)

In addition to "unmasking" that can occur among patients with undiagnosed TB who start ART, it is also common for ART-naïve patients with known TB on antituberculosis therapy to experience worsening of TB-related symptoms when ART is started, or IRIS. After other potential causes of clinical worsening, such as treatment failure related to drug-resistant disease or new opportunistic infection, have been ruled out, IRIS can be managed with prednisone given at a dose of 1.5 mg/kg per day for 2 weeks followed by 0.75 mg/kg per day for 2 weeks [49]. In most cases, ART can be continued without interruption.

6.2   Pediatric Tuberculosis

6.2.1   Epidemiology of Pediatric Tuberculosis

Accurate accounting of pediatric TB is challenging due to the difficulty in confirming the diagnosis and the underappreciation of pediatric TB as a public health issue by TB programs given the child's rare ability to transmit disease. The World Health Organization (WHO) estimates that approximately one million children developed incident TB in 2015, with 140,000 deaths [2]. Modeling studies suggest this likely underestimates pediatric TB disease, as WHO methods account for underreporting, but not underdiagnosis [50].

Worldwide, HIV has fueled the TB epidemic, resulting in both an increased number of TB cases worldwide and also a shift in the epidemic to women of childbearing age, putting young children at significant risk. Additionally, infants diagnosed with HIV are 24 times more likely to develop TB [51]. Though likely underreported, HIV coinfection accounts for only 2 % of US-born and 4 % of foreign-born pediatric tuberculosis [52]. Even still, HIV testing is an important part of the evaluation of TB in all ages.

TB incidence in the USA has dramatically fallen for both adults and children over the last 60 years due to improvements in diagnosis, treatment, and public health measures, including aggressive contact tracing and directly observed therapy. Since 1993, pediatric TB incidence in the USA has fallen from 2.9 to 0.9 cases per 100,000 [53]. Because children acquire TB from adults, it follows that those children at risk have similar epidemiology to those adults with TB. Of pediatric TB cases in the USA, 31 % are among foreign-born children [52]. The most common countries of origin are Mexico, the Philippines, India, Vietnam, and China [53]. The highest rates of TB are among children under 5 years of age (30/100,000), but the greatest discrepancy in incidence between US-born and foreign-born individuals is for adolescents (age 13–17 years). Foreign-born adolescents have an 18-fold higher risk of TB than their US-born counterparts, and incidence in this group has not improved from 1994 to 2007 [52]. Among those US-born patients, 66 % had a foreign-born parent, but 25 % had no international connection through family or residence [54]. Ethnic and racial minorities also are disproportionately affected, with Black (23 %), Asian (20 %), and Latino (29 %) individuals representing a large portion of cases in the USA [53]. Other risk factors include those children exposed to correctional facilities, homelessness, and HIV [53].

The burden of drug-resistant tuberculosis is growing worldwide. Though children do not often contribute to transmission of drug-resistant tuberculosis, they can acquire it. In the USA, INH resistance and MDR and XDR tuberculosis were similar in proportion to adults.

6.2.2   Pathophysiology of Pediatric Tuberculosis

Natural History of Pediatric Tuberculosis

Most pediatric TB is paucibacillary, which has significant implications for transmission, diagnosis, treatment, and the development of drug resistance. Children less than 5 years of age also have relatively immature immune systems and, therefore, have not only a higher risk of disease progression after primary infection but also more commonly present with severe, disseminated disease including both miliary TB and TB meningitis (TBM). This risk is more prominent at younger ages. Among infants, 30–40 % develop pulmonary TB and 10–20 % develop disseminated TB. Among young children, the risk of disseminated disease decreases until 5 years of age when the risk is 2 % [55].

Primary infection occurs when inhaled bacilli reach the distal airways and establish a parenchymal (Ghon) focus of infection. Unable to be contained by the innate immune system, bacilli drain into either perihilar or paratracheal lymph nodes. Together, the Ghon focus and the TB lymphadenitis are referred to as "primary infection." This can occur in up to 50–70 % of children, some of whom will remain asymptomatic, with abnormalities that resolve spontaneously without intervention. Occult hematogenous spread is thought to occur during the establishment of this infection and, in small children, leads to disseminated TB as early as 1 month later. The Ghon focus of infection itself can become uncontained, resulting in parenchymal destruction and cavity formation. More commonly, disease progression stems from unresolved lymph node disease. Lymph nodes can compress a child's relatively compressible airways or extend to other thoracic structures, including the pleura and pericardium. Consolidations are typically unilateral and can be patchy or involve an entire lobe. Caseating pneumonia is also associated with hematogenous spread and TBM in children under 2 years old. Bilateral disease is more commonly associated with miliary disease. Pleural disease and cavitation are less common in young children [55].

Peri-pubescent adolescents are also at high risk of TB, with 10–20 % developing disease after primary infection. Reactivation disease also occurs in this age group. Children older than 7 years of age and adolescents can develop pulmonary disease with high bacillary loads and cavitation. Their symptoms are more akin to adult disease [55].

Pediatric Transmission

Children generally do not transmit TB because of the paucibacillary nature of their disease and the lack of forceful
cough with subsequent inability to generate droplet nuclei
[56–58]. When school-aged children and adolescents have
adult-type disease, with pneumonia or cavitation on chest
radiography, they, too, can spread TB.

6.2.3   Presentations of Pediatric Tuberculosis

Pulmonary Tuberculosis

The signs and symptoms of pediatric intrathoracic disease
can be subtle. Infants often present with nonproductive
cough and mild tachypnea. Many infants will also present
with failure to thrive. Fever, night sweats, anorexia, and
irritability are less common. While respiratory distress is
rare, wheezes, crackles, and hepatosplenomegaly are often
found on examination. Localized wheezes and decreased
breath sounds can also occur in the setting of bronchial
obstruction [59, 60]. Persistent fever without a source is an
important presentation of TB in children and should be
included in the differential diagnosis of fever of unknown
origin.

Cervical Lymphadenitis

Tuberculous lymphadenitis is the most common form of
extrapulmonary TB in children. The presentation is subacute
and first presents with a firm lymph node(s) that later
becomes fixed and matted, most commonly cervical. Over
time, a violaceous skin discoloration overlying a fluctuant
node followed by spontaneous drainage and sinus tract formation develops [61–63]. In low-incidence settings, it is both
important and challenging to distinguish this from more common nontuberculous mycobacterial infections.

Tuberculous Meningitis

TBM is the most severe manifestation of pediatric TB and most commonly presents in children under 5 years of age. Early diagnosis and therapy are essential in preventing morbidity and mortality, but diagnosis remains challenging given that the early signs of disease – fever, listlessness, and vomiting – are nonspecific [64, 65]. Without early treatment and anti-inflammatory medications, increased intracranial pressure and cerebral vasculitis can cause reduced levels of consciousness along with progressive and irreversible neurologic deficits [65].

Congenital Tuberculosis

Congenital tuberculosis develops when a pregnant woman develops hematogenous dissemination of TB. Transmission occurs via the fetal circulation or as a result of inhalation or ingestion of amniotic fluid [66]. Those infections occurring through the fetal circulation commonly result in a hepatic primary focus. Infants present at 2–3 weeks of age with non-specific symptoms including fever, hepatosplenomegaly, lymphadenopathy, respiratory distress, lethargy, irritability, and papular skin lesions [67]. True congenital transmission is rare; more commonly transmission is postpartum from a close contact to a highly susceptible infant.

6.2.4   Diagnosis of Pediatric Tuberculosis

Microbiologic Testing

Given the paucibacillary nature of pediatric TB and the difficulty in obtaining sputum from children, it is often challenging to confirm the diagnosis with laboratory testing [68–72]. Three consecutive early morning gastric lavage specimens, to obtain swallowed sputum, have long been considered the standard of care. Because the specimens are often low yield, clinicians may forego obtaining invasive specimens, using the clinical picture and supportive imaging to diagnose pulmonary TB. Even still, considerable effort should be made to confirm the diagnosis microbiologically and determine drug susceptibility. When the clinical picture is unclear, the child's TB contact is unknown, or there are epidemiological risk factors for drug resistance, a more aggressive approach to obtaining a microbiological diagnosis is even more critical.

Collection of multiple specimens and multiple specimen types remains the optimal approach in confirming the diagnosis [71, 73, 74]. Induced sputum has been shown to be safe and effective, proving to be nearly equivalent to three gastric lavages in sicker hospitalized patients [75], but has had variable results in the ambulatory setting [71, 74]. Table 6.1 shows the sensitivity of gastric lavage and induced sputum specimens. Though widely available, smear microscopy has low sensitivity with a less than 10 % yield. GeneXpert™ is significantly more sensitive than smear and provides information on the most common rifampin resistance-conferring mutations. Even still, GeneXpert misses as much as 40 % of pediatric TB [81]. Culture remains the gold standard, and while sensitivities vary widely, most studies report a 15–30 % yield [70, 77, 81].

There is ongoing research to evaluate alternative patient samples including nasopharyngeal aspirate and stool [78, 83]. Urine tests for LAM are sensitive in adults with advanced HIV disease, but have low sensitivity and specificity in children [84].

The Role of Imaging

Chest radiograph findings in pediatric TB widely vary. The most common findings include lymphadenopathy, often with central necrosis, and airspace disease, with or without cavitations. Miliary disease presents with disseminated nodules [85]. Interreader discordance is high among radiologists, pediatricians, and family doctors [82, 86]. Computed tomography (CT) may be useful in better defining the extent and

Table 6.1 Diagnostic yields from clinical specimens in children with pulmonary tuberculosis

	Gastric lavage		Induced sputum		Nasopharyngeal aspirate	
	One specimen	Multiple specimens	One specimen	Multiple specimens	One specimen	Multiple specimens
Smear	2.2 % (1.4–6.9) [68, 71, 75, 77]	7.0 % (2.3–10.4) [68, 71, 75]	5.2 % (3.5–8.0) [71, 75, 78–80]	6.7 % (5.3–10) [71, 75, 78, 80]	3.9 % [78]	2.7 % (1.4–4.0) [68, 78]
GeneXpertTM	4.2 % [77]		10.4 % (3.9–12.6) [70, 78, 80, 81]	11.4 % (5.2–15.1) [70, 78, 80, 81]	5.8 % (2.3–9.2) [78, 81]	7.0 % (3.6–10.4) [78, 81]
Culture	8.5 % (6.1–42.0) [68, 71, 74, 75, 77]	15.0 % (3.1–66.0) [68, 71, 72, 74, 82]	15.0 % (3.0–38.0) [70, 71, 74, 75, 78–80]	18.3 % (15.1–55.0) [19, 20, 23, 24, 28, 61, 70, 71, 74, 75, 78, 80]	11.4 % [78]	8.8 % (5.5–12.1) [68, 78]

Adapted from Salazar-Austin et al. [76]

anatomical location of disease – lymphadenopathy, parenchymal lesions, and complications of TB including airway narrowing [85]. While CT scan is often deferred in small children due to the perceived risk of radiation, new customized pediatric protocols allow for lower radiation exposure equivalent to 3 months of natural background exposure [87].

6.2.5   Treatment of Pediatric Tuberculosis

Principles of Pediatric Tuberculosis Therapy

The principles of therapy are the same for children as they are for adults. While one should always strive for microbiologic confirmation, this may not always be possible, and lack of confirmation should not prevent initiating treatment in the proper clinical setting. Treatment regimens should initially be based on the source case's drug susceptibility results. When the source case is unknown or their drug susceptibilities are unavailable, the local epidemiology, the patient's personal history of TB, and the source cases' adherence and treatment history are all relevant in assessing the likelihood of transmitted or acquired drug resistance. When resistance is possible or suspected, an aggressive diagnostic approach to obtain a microbiological diagnosis is necessary.

It is suggested that children can be safely and effectively treated with fewer drugs and/or shorter duration than adults, but further clinical trials are needed to define these limits.

Children with known drug-sensitive TB are often treated with a three-drug regimen. Because pediatric TB is paucibacillary and the risk of acquired drug resistance is low, the use of ethambutol is not necessary. This helps to lower pill burden and avoid the risk of optic neuropathy in a small child unable to report early symptoms. The use of ethambutol is indicated in three cases: when the susceptibilities of the child or source case's strains are unknown and the risk of isoniazid mono-resistance is significant, when there is extensive "adult-type" or smear-positive pulmonary disease, and in severe forms of extrapulmonary TB. WHO also uniformly recommends the use of ethambutol in populations with a high prevalence of HIV and INH resistance [88, 89]. Drug doses and formulations of first-line therapy for children are shown in Table 6.2.

Dosing of Anti-TB drugs in Children

Several recent studies have shown that children achieve suboptimal exposures to first-line anti-TB drugs when given the same milligram per kilogram (mg/kg) dose as adults [90–92]. Higher mg/kg doses are now recommended [93]. There has been a long-standing concern regarding the development of optic neuritis in children due to irreversible vision loss following continued use of ethambutol in small children who cannot report early symptoms. However, a thorough review of the literature has demonstrated that ethambutol is safe in children, including infants, at the current recommended dose of 15–25 mg/kg for a 2-month duration [94].

Formulations

Child-friendly, palatable, age-appropriate formulations are essential for achieving optimal drug exposures in children [95]. Pediatric formulations do not exist for many anti-TB drugs and, when they do exist, are not always readily available [96]. New fixed-dose combinations containing the first-line drugs in ratios aligned with current WHO recommendations are expected to come to the market in 2016.

Treatment of Pediatric Drug-Resistant Tuberculosis

Regimens are designed based on the location of infection and the drug resistance pattern of the child or contact case, when susceptibilities are not available for the child. Child-friendly formulations do not exist for many second-line drugs.

TABLE 6.2 Drug therapy for pediatric tuberculosis disease

Drug	Dose	Formulations	Adverse events	Notes
Isoniazid	10 mg/kg (10–15 mg/kg)	Oral tablet (100 mg, 300 mg) Oral solution (50 mg/5 mL) IM solution 100 mg/mL	Hepatotoxicity Peripheral neuropathy Hypersensitivity	Crushed tablets are often better tolerated than liquid isoniazid
Rifampin	15 mg/kg (10–20 mg/kg)	Oral capsule 150 mg, 300 mg Oral suspension 10 mg/mL[a]	Hepatotoxicity "Flu-like" illness with intermittent dosing Hypersensitivity	CYP3A4 inducer Red discoloration of bodily fluids
Pyrazinamide	35 mg/kg (30–40 mg/kg)	Oral tablet 500 mg Oral suspension 100 mg/mL[a]	Hepatotoxicity Hyperuricemia	
Ethambutol	20 mg/kg (15–25 mg/kg)	Oral tablet 100 mg, 400 mg Oral suspension 50 mg/mL[a]	Optic neuritis Hypersensitivity	

[a]Compounding pharmacy must be located

Pediatric infectious disease and tuberculosis specialists should be involved in the development of these regimens.

6.2.6   Prevention of Pediatric Tuberculosis

BCG Vaccine

Bacillus Calmette-Guérin (BCG) is a live attenuated strain of *Mycobacterium bovis* and is currently the only licensed vaccine for TB. The reported efficacy for prevention of pulmonary TB has been inconsistent, ranging from 0 to 80 %. The protective effect against disseminated TB is more evident with meta-analyses showing an efficacy of 86 % [97]. Uncommon complications include localized disease such as abscesses at the site of injection with contiguous spread to the lymph node or bone. Disseminated disease is more uncommon, but immunodeficiency is a risk factor [98]. Recognizing that *M. bovis* is inherently resistant to pyrazinamide, most physicians treat *M. bovis* infection with rifampin, isoniazid, and ethambutol. For serious *M. bovis* disease, some experts recommend longer therapy with higher doses [88].

The risks of BCG vaccine in HIV-infected infants are not well established, though available data suggest that infants are at a several hundredfold increased risk of complications [99]. WHO now recommends a single dose of BCG vaccine for all infants in a highly endemic area who are not known to be or suspected to be HIV infected [88], noting that HIV-infected infants are given BCG prior to their diagnosis of HIV in most highly endemic settings.

Preventive Chemotherapy

Rapid identification of the adult index case and initiation of preventive chemotherapy can be helpful in preventing infection with *M. tuberculosis*. In practice, this may be difficult, as young children, who are the most susceptible to infection, are likely to have been exposed by the time the index case is diagnosed.

Screening for Latent TB Infection (LTBI)

In low-incidence settings, targeted TST is used to identify those children who are most at risk for LTBI. In the USA, risk factors include a contact with either TB disease or LTBI, foreign birth or travel, or interaction with someone who was incarcerated or with someone who was born or has traveled outside the USA. Those children living with HIV should be screened annually with TST. Evaluation of a positive TST result includes clinical evaluation with radiologic imaging. In highly endemic areas, symptom-based screening for active disease has been found to be both safe and effective for the evaluation of child contacts of TB patients [100, 101] and is now recommended by WHO to simplify the process and improve the feasibility by avoiding the need for specialty referral and chest X-ray. Baseline laboratories including liver function tests are not recommended prior to initiation of LTBI treatment [102].

Tuberculin Skin Testing (TST) Versus Interferon-Gamma Release Assays (IGRAs) in Children

Both TST and IGRA are used to detect *M. tuberculosis* infection, but neither of these tests distinguish between infection and disease. Neither test is considered the gold standard for diagnosing TB infection in children. TST requires several crucial steps including precise intradermal injection, time-sensitive patient follow-up 48–72 h postinjection, and accurate reading of transverse induration and not erythema. A positive or negative result is then determined by the patient's risk factors (Table 6.3) [104]. Host factors affecting the sensitivity of TST include young age, poor nutrition, immunosuppression including HIV [105], recent viral infection or recent administration of a live attenuated viral vaccine within 4–6 weeks, recent *M. tuberculosis* infection within the prior 3 months, and disseminated disease. BCG vaccine and nontuberculous mycobacterial (NTM) infection can also cause a false-positive TST, which is difficult to distinguish from LTBI [104].

Table 6.3 Pediatric tuberculin skin test (TST) positivity by risk group

Induration ≥5 mm	Induration ≥10 mm	Induration ≥15 mm
Very high-risk individuals and those with at risk for poor reaction to TST	*High-risk individuals without risk for poor reaction to TST*	*Low-risk individuals*
Clinical evidence of tuberculosis disease	Age <5 years	Children ≥5 years old without risk factors
Contact with an infectious tuberculosis case	Foreign born from high-prevalence countries	
Fibrotic changes on CXR consistent with prior tuberculosis	Foreign travel to a high-prevalence countries	
Immunosuppressed including HIV	Children and adolescents with frequent exposure to high-risk adults (HIV+, homeless, illicit drug users, residents of prisons, healthcare facilities, or nursing homes)	
Immunosuppressive drug therapy including corticosteroids (>15 mg/day or duration >1 month) and TNF-α antagonists	Medical risk factors: diabetes mellitus, Hodgkin disease, lymphoma, chronic renal failure, malnutrition	
	Children and adolescents exposed to adults in high-risk categories	

Adapted from [103]

TABLE 6.4 Choosing TST versus IGRA in children

Reasons to choose TST	Reasons to choose IGRA
<5 years old regardless of BCG vaccination	Any child who is >5 years old
Multiple attempts at IGRA with indeterminate results	>5 years and BCG vaccinated
IGRA too expensive, lack of insurance	Those >5 years who are less likely to return for TST reading
HIV positive	

Adapted from [103]

IGRAs are expensive but do not require a return visit, and they are more specific for *M. tuberculosis* than TST. IGRA does not cross-react with BCG or most nontuberculous mycobacteria. Sensitivity is poor in children under 5 years of age, and IGRA testing is, therefore, not recommended for this age group [103]; however, when positive, the result is reliable. Table 6.4 describes those situations where either TST or IGRA is preferred. Expert opinion should be sought if testing is needed in someone who was recently vaccinated with BCG.

Treatment of LTBI in Children

IPT has long been known to be highly efficacious in children [106, 107], and the duration of the prophylactic effect is likely to be lifelong, particularly in areas of low TB endemicity [108]. Several regimens [109, 110] have been evaluated, and specific dosing information for children is available in Table 6.5. Regimen choice is dependent on source case's drug susceptibility, the child's comorbidities, the drug interactions, the cost, and the desired time frame of therapy. Clinical trials have shown increased efficacy with shorter regimens attributed to improved adherence and completion of therapy [111]. Only 12-month isoniazid regimens have been evaluated in children, but six- and 9-month regimens are widely accepted and are recommended by the Joint Tuberculosis Committee and the American Academy of Pediatrics, respectively [112, 113].

Children often tolerate LTBI therapy better than adults. Hepatotoxicity has been reported to be less than 2 % with traditional IPT regimens [114–116], and there has been no reported increase in severe reactions with any of the regimens listed in Table 6.5. LTBI treatment with rifapentine and isoniazid may be especially attractive in children, as dosing is once weekly, and the total number of doses is 12 [109, 117]. Given the overall low risk of hepatotoxicity in children receiving TB prophylaxis, routine laboratory monitoring is not needed for any of the recommended regimens.

Preventive chemoprophylaxis for children who are close contacts of patients with multidrug-resistant TB is described in Sect. 6.3.7.

6.3   Drug-Resistant Tuberculosis

6.3.1   Definitions

Multidrug-resistant tuberculosis (MDR-TB) is resistant to the most effective first-line agents: isoniazid and rifampin. Extensively, drug-resistant tuberculosis (XDR-TB) is resistant to isoniazid and rifampin plus any of the fluoroquinolones and at least one second-line injectable agent (kanamycin, amikacin, or capreomycin).

6.3.2   Epidemiology of Drug-Resistant Tuberculosis

DR-TB is becoming increasingly prevalent worldwide and presents a serious threat to global TB control. WHO estimates that 3.3 % of new TB cases and 20 % of previously treated TB cases worldwide are MDR-TB. About 10 % of

TABLE 6.5 Pediatric regimens for treatment of LTBI

Chemoprophylaxis regimen	Dose	Interval	Duration	Hepatotoxicity	Side effects	Notes
Isoniazid	10–15 mg/kg	Daily	6–12 months	<1 %	Peripheral neuropathy (rare), GI upset, rash (2 %)	9-month regimen is referred regimen by AAP for immunocompetent children, WHO recommends 6 months
Isoniazid	20–30 mg/kg	Twice weekly	6–12 months			DOT is strongly recommended
Rifampin	10–20 mg/kg	Daily	4 months	<2 %	GI upset, rash (2 %), thrombocytopenia 3.4 %	
Isoniazid and rifampin	Isoniazid: 10–15 mg/kg Rifampin: 10–15 mg/kg	Daily	3 months	1–2 %		

(continued)

TABLE 6.5 (continued)

Chemoprophylaxis regimen	Dose	Interval	Duration	Hepatotoxicity	Side effects	Notes
Isoniazid and rifapentine	INH: <12 years old 25 mg/kg ≥12 years old 15 mg/kg (max 900 mg for all ages) Rifapentine: 10–14 kg: 300 mg 14.1–25 kg: 450 mg 25.1–32 kg: 600 mg 32.1–50 kg: 750 mg >50 kg: 900 mg	Once weekly	3 months, 12 doses	0.4 %	Rifapentine: GI upset, rash	>2 years old DOT is strongly recommended

MDR-TB have further resistance and can be classified as XDR-TB [2].

Despite substantial progress in the development of rapid diagnostic tests for detection of DR-TB, WHO estimates that just 41 % of patients with MDR-TB worldwide were diagnosed in 2014 [2]. Furthermore, there continues to be a significant delay between diagnosis and initiation of treatment in much of the world, though MDR initiations increased by 14 % worldwide in 2014. Therapeutic options are limited and costly and treatment is poorly efficacious and prolonged, and these factors may contribute to continued spread of drug-resistant TB in endemic areas.

In the USA, about 10 % of TB cases are resistant to isoniazid, and less than 2 % of TB cases are MDR. Greater than 80 % of cases of primary MDR (MDR-TB among patients with no previous history of TB treatment) are in foreign-born persons. There are a small number of XDR-TB cases in the USA each year [53]. WHO reports that the following countries account for about 75 % of DR-TB: India, China, the Russian Federation, Eastern European countries, and South Africa [2]. Long-term travelers to endemic countries have substantial risk, similar to that of the local population [118]. DR-TB should be considered and sought among patients with suspected TB for whom there is no clear contact with drug-sensitive TB or among individuals with a history of foreign travel.

6.3.3   Primary and Acquired Resistance

Drug resistance can be primary or acquired. That is, someone may have primary infection transmitted directly from a person with MDR-TB infection, or a patient may have a history of prior drug-susceptible TB with subsequent development of acquired drug resistance. Despite the presence of multiple mutations, MDR- and XDR-TB strains appear to be quite fit and can be transmitted as readily as drug-sensitive TB [119–121]. How acquired resistance develops is incompletely understood. Traditionally, it was thought that poor adherence led to periods of effective monotherapy with regimens comprised of drugs with different half-lives [122]. However, direct evidence that treatment default and poor adherence are major factors leading to acquired resistance and MDR-TB is lacking. Newer experiments and clinical data suggest that there is significant pharmacokinetic variability among patients taking standard doses of anti-TB drugs, and low exposures among patients who are fully adherent with TB therapy may contribute substantially toward the development of resistance [123, 124].

6.3.4   Transmission Risk

Traditionally, in the case of drug-susceptible TB, after 2 weeks of first-line therapy, a patient is generally considered to be noninfectious, irrespective of smear and culture conversion, and respiratory isolation is discontinued. With limited supporting data, this "2-week rule" has become a standard in infection control. There are no data specific to MDR-TB, but infection control programs have been more conservative with MDR-TB, requiring smear or culture conversion before discontinuing respiratory isolation. Not unexpectedly, those with undiagnosed drug resistance treated with empiric, but suboptimal, regimens are infectious for a prolonged period of time [125]. Almost certainly the period of infectiousness varies from regimen to regimen, and by the extent of disease, but data to inform infection control practices are lacking.

6.3.5   Diagnostics for Drug Resistance

Clinically, DR-TB should be suspected in the setting of (1) a known contact with DR-TB, (2) travel to a DR-TB endemic area, or (3) persistent signs and symptoms of TB, ongoing microbiological positivity, or worsening radiology in the setting of generally effective first-line therapy.

Phenotypic Testing

The Middlebrook 7H10 agar proportion method is the gold standard for susceptibility testing for *M. tuberculosis*. This testing is available at a small number of reference laboratories including state laboratories and the CDC. Laborious, this method requires at least 2–3 weeks of culture and reports only susceptibility to one or two critical concentrations of drug. These critical concentrations are largely historical and may not reflect achievable drug concentrations or predict clinical failure [126, 127].

The Sensititre MYCOTB plate utilizes liquid culture and tests a range of drug concentrations to reliably determine not only susceptibility, but a more precise MIC in just 10–14 days. Though not yet standard in every mycobacteriology laboratory, a more precise MIC may allow for the construction of more durable regimens to prevent the acquired resistance [128, 129].

Pyrazinamide susceptibility testing is challenging because of the need for acidic culture media (which may itself contribute to poor growth) and the observation that large inocula may decrease pyrazinamide's efficacy, leading to a false-positive result for resistance [130, 131]. Liquid culture is recommended but remains imperfect.

Genotypic Tests

Mutations in *pncA* have been associated with resistance to pyrazinamide [132]. Likewise, mutations in other genes correlate with resistance to other first- and second-line antituberculous drugs (Table 6.6). While genotypic drug susceptibility testing (DST) can be faster than traditional phenotypic DST and can guide therapeutic decisions in a more timely manner, results of genotypic and phenotypic DST are not always concordant, and in these cases, phenotypic DST remains the gold standard.

First recommended by WHO in 2010, and approved by the FDA in 2013, Xpert® MTB/RIF (Cepheid, Sunnyvale, USA) is an automated nucleic-acid amplification test that provides

TABLE 6.6 Most common mutations associated with resistance to first- and second-line antituberculous drugs

Antituberculous Drug	Mutation	Likelihood of conferring resistance	Notes
Rifampicin	*rpoB*(Ser521Leu)	100 % isolates are thought to be resistant	Account for >95 % of rifampin resistance
Isoniazid	*katG* (Ser315Thr)	High level resistance: 100 % isolates are thought to be resistant	Together, these mutations account for ~80 % of studied isolates resistant to INH
	inhA (position 15 of INH promoter)	Low level resistance: High-dose isoniazid may overcome resistance	
Pyrazinamide	*pncA (Asp12Glu)*	Likely	No optimal gold standard for phenotypic resistance testing to confirm genotypic resistance
Ethambutol	*embB* (Met306Ile)	Resistance is likely but not certain	
	embB (Gly406)		
Fluoroquinolone	*gryA* (Asp94Gly)	100 % isolates are thought to be resistant	
Aminoglycoside: Amikacin Kanamycin Capreomycin	*rrs* (A1401G), Also C1402T, G1484T??? *Eis* (promoter) *tlyA* (entire ORF)	No single or set of mutations reliably predict phenotypic sensitivity to all three drugs	Streptomycin has been poorly studied and particular mutations conferring resistance are unknown
Ethionamide	*inhA*	High-level resistance	

rapid, accurate, and simultaneous diagnosis of both *M. tuberculosis* complex disease and rifampin resistance [133]. In the USA, this test is increasingly available in state health laboratories. Initially, the test was only validated for use with pulmonary specimens, but in 2013, WHO expanded recommendations for use of this test to include multiple other matrices, with appropriate processing of samples – CSF, pleural biopsy, lymph tissue or aspirate, and gastric aspirate in children [134].

Local epidemiology should always inform decision-making. Thirty percent (30 %) of MDR-TB strains in Swaziland have rifampin resistance that lies outside those regions of the *rpoB* gene detected by Xpert® [135]. Next-generation Xpert® improves sensitivity in both the detection of tuberculosis DNA and rifampin resistance [136].

6.3.6 Treatment of DR-Tuberculosis

Principles of Treatment

The principles of treatment for DR-TB are similar to those for treatment of DS-TB, though regimens must be built with drugs that are less efficacious, more toxic, and, in some cases, very expensive. Treatment regimens generally include at least four drugs to which the patient's isolate is expected to be sensitive, based on in vitro DST of the infecting strain plus the patient's treatment history, drug susceptibility information from the source case, and local epidemiologic data. Five drugs are often used for XDR-TB. With few therapeutic options and localized disease, surgery may be a useful adjunctive treatment [137].

Drug Regimens

The WHO has recently revised how it categorizes drugs for treatment of DR-TB. First line medications include rifampicin, isoniazid, pyrazinamide and ethambutol. Second line agents are grouped into 4 categories, A through D (Tables 6.7 and 6.8). Group A includes fluoroquinolones with anti-tuberculous activity, Group B consists of injectable agents, generally a

TABLE 6.7 World Health Organization (WHO) recommended medicines for the treatment of MDR-TB [138]

Group	Drugs	
A. Fluoroquinolones		Levofloxacin
		Moxifloxacin
		Gatifloxacin
B. Second-line injectable agents		Amikacin
		Capreomycin
		Kanamycin
		(Streptomycin)
C. Other core second-line agents		Ethionamide/Prothionamide
		Cycloserine/Terizidone
		Linezolid
		Clofazimine
D. Add-on agents (not part of the core MDR-TB regimen)	D1	Pyrazinamide
		Ethambutol
		High-dose isoniazid
	D2	Bedaquiline
		Delamanid
	D3	p-Aminosalicyclic acid
		Imipenem–cilastatin
		Meropenem
		Amoxicillin–clavulanate
		(Thioacetazone)

TABLE 6.8 Second-line anti-TB drugs

Drug	Adult dose	Pediatric dose	Side effects	Notes
Pyrazinamide	1–2 g daily based on weight	30–40 mg/kg	Hepatitis arthritis	Pyrazinamide should be included as a fifth agent
Ethambutol	25 mg/kg, (range 8–1600 g)	20–25 mg/kg for DR-TB	Optic neuritis GI disturbance	May be used, but should be included as a fifth agent
Fluoroquinolone	Levo: 500–1000 mg daily Moxi: 400 mg daily	Oflox: 15–20 mg/kg Levo: 7.5–10 mg/kg (BID if <5 yo) Moxi: 7.5–10 mg/kg (for children >12)	Sleep disturbance GI disturbance Arthritis Peripheral neuropathy	When susceptible, a FQ is advisable
Amikacin Kanamycin Capreomycin Streptomycin	A, K, C, S: 15–30 mg/kg (max 1g)	A: 15–22.5 mg/kg K: 15–30 mg/kg C: 15–30 mg/kg S: 15–20 mg/kg	Oto- and vestibular toxicity Nephrotoxicity	Daily at first, can decrease to thrice weekly 2–4 months after sputum conversion
Ethionamide	500–750 mg divided 1–2 times daily (max 1 g/day)	15–20 mg/kg	GI disturbance Metallic taste Hypothyroidism Hepatitis	inhA mutation confers cross resistance to ethionamide
Prothionamide		15–20 mg/kg	Same as ethionamide	Never in combination with ethionamide
Cycloserine	Ramp up to 500–750 mg divided BID (max 1g)	15–20 mg/kg	Neuropsychiatric effects Seizures Rash	Preferable to PAS With vitamin B6

(continued)

TABLE 6.8 (continued)

Drug	Adult dose	Pediatric dose	Side effects	Notes
Terizidone	15–20 mg/kg		Same as cycloserine	Never in combination with cycloserine
PAS	8–12 g/d divided 2–3 times daily	150 mg/kg	GI intolerance Hypothyroidism Hepatitis Hypersensitivity Thrombocytopenia	When cycloserine cannot be used
Clofazimine	100 mg daily	3–5 mg/kg *	Skin discoloration Ichthyosis Severe GI effects	Acceptability of the skin discoloration that will occur may vary by setting
Linezolid	600 mg daily, then dose reduction to 300 mg	10 mg/kg BID	Bone marrow suppression Peripheral neuropathy Optic neuropathy Pancreatitis	Promising, but significantly limited by neuropathy and bone marrow suppression. Dose reduction to 300 mg often required
Delamanid	100 mg BID	–	QT prolongation	Pediatric dosing not yet established but studies in progress to do so
Bedaquiline	400 mg daily for 14 days then 200 mg thrice weekly	–	QT prolongation	Pediatric dosing not yet established but studies in progress to do so

staple of DR-TB multidrug regimens, but plagued by serious side effects such as renal injury and hearing loss. Group C consists of other core second-line agents. Finally add-on agents are included in Group D. D1 agents are first-line drugs, D2 includes new drugs, and D3 primarily consists of drugs for which the anti-TB activity was previously uncertain, though understanding of these drugs' potential contribution to DR-TB regimens is evolving.

DR-TB regimens should include pyrazinamide along with a fluoroquinolone (Group A), an injectable agent (Group B, except in children with non-severe disease), and two Group C agents. Group C drugs are ordered by preference given available evidence, experience and tolerability. They should be chosen based on local susceptibility patterns, consideration of the side effects profile (and a given patient's comorbidities), and availability. Group C includes ethionamide or prothionamide (assuming no *inhA* promoter mutations), cycloserine or terizidone, linezolid, and clofazimine [139, 140]. High-dose INH and/or ethambutol should be added to further strengthen the regimen, depending on what is known about the patient's isolate's susceptibility pattern (Group D1).

If a 5-drug regimen cannot be composed using drugs in groups A–D1, bedaquiline or delamanid (Group D2) can be added; these drugs may be especially useful among those patients with isolates resistant to fluoroquinolones, injectable agents, or both or who cannot tolerate standard MDR-TB drugs [141, 142]. Additionally, Group D3 drugs can be added to bring the total to five active drugs. P-aminosalicylic acid is active against tuberculosis, but significant GI upset limits its use. Thioacetazone should only be given to confirmed HIV-negative patients. MDR-TB regimens include an 8-month intensive phase followed by a 12-month continuation phase.

Despite a relative paucity of data, the WHO announced in May 2016 a standardized short course MDR-TB regimen with the hope that lowered costs and fewer losses in follow up may enable a more feasible and effective regimen for MDR TB worldwide. The shorter regimen of 9–12 months applies to pulmonary MDR-TB patients, regardless of HIV status, who have not had prolonged (>1 month) exposure to second line agents, including fluoroquinolones and injectable agents, where resistance to these agents has been excluded or is highly unlikely. Patients who are pregnant or who have extrapulmonary TB are not eligible for the shorter course therapy. This regimen consists of a standard regimen of Kanamycin, moxifloxacin, prothionamide, clofazimine, pyrazinamide and high-dose isoniazid for 4–6 months of an intensive phase followed by a 5 month continuation phase consisting of moxifloacin, clofazimine, pyrazinamide and ethambutol.

Children remain eligible for shorter course therapy despite exclusion from all previous clinical trials evaluating shorter course therapy, because there is no plausible pathophysiologic explanation for why short course therapy would be less efficacious in children than adults. For non-severe paucibacilliary pediatric disease, injectable agents can be excluded from a child's regimen [138].

Construction of any DR-TB regimen should include guidance from an infectious disease specialist familiar with TB therapy. For isoniazid-monoresistant TB, a fluoroquinolone such as moxifloxacin or levofloxacin can be substituted for isoniazid, based on indirect evidence [143, 144].

Treatment duration

Little is known about appropriate durations of therapy. Based predominantly on observational studies, WHO recommends that patients with MDR-TB receive intensive phase therapy for at least 4 months after culture conversion and for a minimum of 8 months, followed by continuation phase therapy in which the injectable agent is generally dropped. The total duration of therapy should be at least 20–24 months [145]. The short-course treatment regimen above is given for 9–12 months. Clinical studies evaluating a similar regimen – a late-generation fluoroquinolone, clofazimine, ethambutol, and pyrazinamide throughout treatment supplemented with an injectable agent, ethionamide or prothionamide, and high-dose isoniazid during the 4–6-month intensive phase – have resulted in success rates as high as 85–90 % [146, 147]. Clinical trials formally comparing this shorter "Bangladesh regimen" to standard MDR-TB regimens are ongoing.

Safety and tolerability

MDR-TB treatment regimens are poorly tolerated and have significant, often treatment-limiting toxicities. The injectable agents cause ototoxicity, which can be irreversible. Ethionamide and prothionamide cause dose-limiting gastro-intestinal toxicity, while cycloserine and terizidone result in serious CNS side effects. Linezolid causes peripheral neuropathy and bone marrow suppression. Clofazimine causes skin discoloration. Hypersensitivity, ophthalmologic toxicity, liver injury, drug-induced lupus, thyroid dysregulation, QT interval prolongation, and electrolyte disturbances are other common side effects with multidrug MDR- or XDR-TB regimens. Careful clinical and laboratory monitoring of patients by trained specialists is of the utmost importance.

Treatment outcomes

Reported treatment outcomes for DR-TB have been significantly inferior to those of drug-susceptible TB, with worsening outcomes as the number of drugs to which the TB is resistant increases. Meta-analyses have demonstrated favorable MDR-TB outcomes, including cure and treatment completion, in only 54–70 % of those treated [148–151]. In initial reports of XDR-TB occurring among patients with high rates of HIV coinfection in Tugela Ferry in 2006, mortality was nearly 100 % [152]. Since that time, observational studies have demonstrated improved outcomes with 43 % having favorable outcomes in a meta-analysis [153] and a range of 12–66 % favorable outcomes in observational studies [154–159]. WHO's 2015 global TB report estimates that the treatment success rate remains low at 50 % for MDR patients and 26 % for XDR patients. WHO cites health system weaknesses, lack of availability of effective regimens, and other treatment challenges for unacceptably low cure rates.

6.3.7   Preventive Chemotherapy

Currently, no chemotherapy regimens have proven efficacy for preventing development of MDR-TB among contacts of MDR-TB cases. Prospective cohort studies in children exposed to MDR-TB and treated with multidrug preventive chemotherapeutic regimens have shown these regimens to be well tolerated and seemingly efficacious [160]. In the setting of two simultaneous MDR-TB outbreaks in Micronesia, prophylactic regimens of moxifloxacin or levofloxacin with or without ethambutol (depending on the susceptibility pattern of the most likely infecting strain) were given to adult and child contacts of MDR-TB patients [161]. The regimens were well tolerated and appeared to be effective in this relatively small group of patients. Definitive trials to inform the content and duration of regimens for MDR-TB prophylaxis are needed.

References

1. UNAIDS Joint United Nations Programme on HIV/AIDS. UNAIDS Global Report 2013; 2013.
2. WHO. Global tuberculosis report 2015. World Health Organization, Geneva; 2015. http://www.who.int/tb/publications/global_report/en/. Last accessed March 11, 2016.
3. Sonnenberg P, Glynn J, Fielding K, Murray J, Godfrey-Faussett P, Shearer S. How soon after infection with HIV does the risk of tuberculosis start to increase? A retrospective cohort study in South African gold miners. J Infect Dis. 2005;191(2):150–8.
4. Wood R, Maartens G, Lombard C. Risk factors for developing tuberculosis in HIV-1-infected adults from communities with a low or very high incidence of tuberculosis. J Acquir Immune Defic Syndr. 2000;23(1):75–80.
5. Selwyn P, Hartel D, Lewis V, Schoenbaum E, Vermund S, Klein R. A prospective study of the risk of tuberculosis among intravenous drug users with human immunodeficiency virus infection. N Engl J Med. 1989;320(9):545–50.
6. Centers for Disease Control and Prevention (CDC). TB and HIV Coinfection. CDC Factsheet. https://www.cdc.gov/tb/topic/tbhivcoinfection/default.htm. Accessed March 11, 2015.

7. Temprano Anrs Study Group, Danel C, Moh R, Gabillard D, Badje A, Le Carrou J, et al. A trial of early antiretrovirals and isoniazid preventive therapy in Africa. N Engl J Med. 2015;373(9):808–22.

8. Suthar AB, Lawn SD, del Amo J, Getahun H, Dye C, Sculier D, et al. Antiretroviral therapy for prevention of tuberculosis in adults with HIV: a systematic review and meta-analysis. PLoS Med. 2012;9(7):e1001270.

9. Severe P, Juste MA, Ambroise A, Eliacin L, Marchand C, Apollon S, et al. Early versus standard antiretroviral therapy for HIV-infected adults in Haiti. N Engl J Med. 2010;363(3):257–65.

10. Briggs MA, Emerson C, Modi S, Taylor NK. Use of isoniazid preventive therapy for tuberculosis prophylaxis among people living with HIV/AIDS: a review of the literature. J Acquir Immune Defic Syndr. 2015;68 Suppl 3:S297–305.

11. Golub JE, Pronyk P, Mohapi L, Thsabangu N, Moshabela M, Struthers H, et al. Isoniazid preventive therapy, HAART and tuberculosis risk in HIV-infected adults in South Africa: a prospective cohort. AIDS. 2009;23(5):631–6.

12. Jones JL, Hanson DL, Dworkin MS, DeCock KM. Adult/Adolescent Spectrum of HIVDG. HIV-associated tuberculosis in the era of highly active antiretroviral therapy. The Adult/Adolescent Spectrum of HIV Disease Group. Int J Tuberc Lung Dis. 2000;4(11):1026–31.

13. Golub JE, Saraceni V, Cavalcante SC, Pacheco AG, Moulton LH, King BS, et al. The impact of antiretroviral therapy and isoniazid preventive therapy on tuberculosis incidence in HIV-infected patients in Rio de Janeiro Brazil. AIDS. 2007;21(11): 1441–8.

14. Trajman A, Steffen R, Menzies D. Interferon-gamma release assays versus tuberculin skin testing for the diagnosis of latent tuberculosis infection: an overview of the evidence. Pulm Med. 2013;2013:601737.

15. Rangaka MX, Wilkinson KA, Glynn JR, Ling D, Menzies D, Mwansa-Kambafwile J, et al. Predictive value of interferon-gamma release assays for incident active tuberculosis: a systematic review and meta-analysis. Lancet Infect Dis. 2012;12(1):45–55.

16. Ayele HT, Mourik MS, Debray TP, Bonten MJ. Isoniazid prophylactic therapy for the prevention of tuberculosis in HIV infected adults: a systematic review and meta-analysis of randomized trials. PLoS One. 2015;10(11):e0142290.

17. Kerkhoff AD, Kranzer K, Samandari T, Nakiyingi-Miiro J, Whalen CC, Harries AD, et al. Systematic review of TST

responses in people living with HIV in under-resourced settings: implications for isoniazid preventive therapy. PLoS One. 2012;7(11):e49928.

18. Hosseinipour M, Bisson G, Miyahara S, Sun X, Moses A, Riviere C, et al. Empiric TB therapy does not decrease early mortality compared to isoniazid preventive therapy in adults with advanced HIV initiating ART: results of ACTG A5274 (REMEMBER study). International AIDS Society Conference. 2015:Abstract MOAB0205LB.

19. Getahun H, Matteelli A, Abubakar I, Aziz MA, Baddeley A, Barreira D, et al. Management of latent Mycobacterium tuberculosis infection: WHO guidelines for low tuberculosis burden countries. Eur Respir J. 2015;46(6):1563–76.

20. Samandari T, Agizew TB, Nyirenda S, Tedla Z, Sibanda T, Shang N, et al. 6-month versus 36-month isoniazid preventive treatment for tuberculosis in adults with HIV infection in Botswana: a randomised, double-blind, placebo-controlled trial. Lancet. 2011;377(9777):1588–98.

21. Swaminathan S, Menon PA, Gopalan N, Perumal V, Santhanakrishnan RK, Ramachandran R, et al. Efficacy of a six-month versus a 36-month regimen for prevention of tuberculosis in HIV-infected persons in India: a randomized clinical trial. PLoS One. 2012;7(12):e47400.

22. Tedla Z, Nguyen ML, Sibanda T, Nyirenda S, Agizew TB, Girde S, et al. Isoniazid-associated hepatitis in adults infected with HIV receiving 36 months of isoniazid prophylaxis in Botswana. Chest. 2015;147(5):1376–84.

23. Sterling TR, Villarino ME, Borisov AS, Shang N, Gordin F, Bliven-Sizemore E, et al. Three months of rifapentine and isoniazid for latent tuberculosis infection. N Engl J Med. 2011;365(23):2155–66.

24. WHO. Guidelines on the management of latent tuberculosis infection. World Health Organization, Geneva; 2015. http://www.who.int/tb/publications/global_report/en/. Last accessed March 11, 2016.

25. Luetkemeyer A, Rosenkranz S, Lu D, Marzan F, Ive P, Hogg E, et al. Relationship between weight, efavirenz exposure and virologic suppression in HIV-infected patients on rifampin-based TB treatment in the ACTG A5221 STRIDE study. Clin Infect Dis. 2013;57(4):586–93.

26. Podany AT, Bao Y, Swindells S, Chaisson RE, Andersen JW, Mwelase T, et al. Efavirenz pharmacokinetics and pharmacody-

namics in HIV-infected persons receiving rifapentine and isoniazid for tuberculosis prevention. Clin Infect Dis. 2015;61(8):1322–7.

27. Weiner M, Egelund EF, Engle M, Kiser M, Prihoda TJ, Gelfond JA, et al. Pharmacokinetic interaction of rifapentine and raltegravir in healthy volunteers. J Antimicrob Chemother. 2014;69(4):1079–85.

28. Jones BE, Young SM, Antoniskis D, Davidson PT, Kramer F, Barnes PF. Relationship of the manifestations of tuberculosis to CD4 cell counts in patients with human immunodeficiency virus infection. Am Rev Respir Dis. 1993;148(5):1292–7.

29. Naing C, Mak JW, Maung M, Wong SF, Kassim AI. Meta-analysis: the association between HIV infection and extrapulmonary tuberculosis. Lung. 2013;191(1):27–34.

30. Meintjes G, Lawn S, Scano F, Maartens G, French M, Worodria W. Tuberculosis-associated immune reconstitution inflammatory syndrome: case definitions for use in resource-limited settings. Lancet Infect Dis. 2008;8(8):516–23.

31. Denkinger CM, Schumacher SG, Boehme CC, Dendukuri N, Pai M, Steingart KR. Xpert MTB/RIF assay for the diagnosis of extrapulmonary tuberculosis: a systematic review and meta-analysis. Eur Respir J. 2014;44(2):435–46.

32. Shah M, Dowdy D, Joloba M, Ssengooba W, Manabe YC, Ellner J, et al. Cost-effectiveness of novel algorithms for rapid diagnosis of tuberculosis in HIV-infected individuals in Uganda. AIDS. 2013;27(18):2883–92.

33. Nakiyingi L, Ssengooba W, Nakanjako D, Armstrong D, Holshouser M, Kirenga B, et al. Predictors and outcomes of mycobacteremia among HIV-infected smear- negative presumptive tuberculosis patients in Uganda. BMC Infect Dis. 2015;15:62. -015-0812-0814.

34. Vernon A, Burman W, Benator D, Khan A, Bozeman L. Acquired rifamycin monoresistance in patients with HIV-related tuberculosis treated with once-weekly rifapentine and isoniazid. Tuberculosis Trials Consortium. Lancet. 1999;353(9167):1843–7.

35. Narendran G, Menon PA, Venkatesan P, Vijay K, Padmapriyadarsini C, Ramesh Kumar S, et al. Acquired rifampicin resistance in thrice-weekly antituberculosis therapy: impact of HIV and anti-retroviral therapy. Clin Infect Dis. 2014;59(12):1798–804.

36. Ahmad Khan F, Minion J, Al-Motairi A, Benedetti A, Harries AD, Menzies D. An updated systematic review and meta-analysis on the treatment of active tuberculosis in patients with HIV infection. Clin Infect Dis. 2012;55(8):1154–63.

37. Abdool Karim SS, Naidoo K, Grobler A, Padayatchi N, Baxter C, Gray A, et al. Timing of initiation of antiretroviral drugs during tuberculosis therapy. N Engl J Med. 2010;362(8):697–706.

38. Abdool Karim SS, Naidoo K, Grobler A, Padayatchi N, Baxter C, Gray AL, et al. Integration of antiretroviral therapy with tuberculosis treatment. N Engl J Med. 2011;365(16):1492–501.

39. Havlir DV, Kendall MA, Ive P, Kumwenda J, Swindells S, Qasba SS, et al. Timing of antiretroviral therapy for HIV-1 infection and tuberculosis. N Engl J Med. 2011;365(16):1482–91.

40. Blanc FX, Sok T, Laureillard D, Borand L, Rekacewicz C, Nerrienet E, et al. Earlier versus later start of antiretroviral therapy in HIV-infected adults with tuberculosis. N Engl J Med. 2011;365(16):1471–81.

41. Mfinanga SG, Kirenga BJ, Chanda DM, Mutayoba B, Mthiyane T, Yimer G, et al. Early versus delayed initiation of highly active antiretroviral therapy for HIV-positive adults with newly diagnosed pulmonary tuberculosis (TB-HAART): a prospective, international, randomised, placebo-controlled trial. Lancet Infect Dis. 2014;14(7):563–71.

42. Insight Start Study Group, Lundgren JD, Babiker AG, Gordin F, Emery S, Grund B, et al. Initiation of antiretroviral therapy in early asymptomatic HIV infection. N Engl J Med. 2015;373(9):795–807.

43. Dooley KE, Flexner C, Andrade AS. Drug interactions involving combination antiretroviral therapy and other anti-infective agents: repercussions for resource-limited countries. J Infect Dis. 2008;198(7):948–61.

44. Grinsztejn B, De Castro N, Arnold V, Veloso VG, Morgado M, Pilotto JH, et al. Raltegravir for the treatment of patients co-infected with HIV and tuberculosis (ANRS 12 180 Reflate TB): a multicentre, phase 2, non-comparative, open-label, randomised trial. Lancet Infect Dis. 2014;14(6):459–67.

45. Dooley K, Sayre P, Borland J, Purdy E, Chen S, Song I, et al. Safety, tolerability, and pharmacokinetics of the HIV integrase inhibitor dolutegravir given twice daily with rifampin or once daily with rifabutin: results of a phase 1 study among healthy subjects. J Acquir Immune Defic Syndr. 2013;62(1):21–7.

46. Naiker S, Connolly C, Wiesner L, Kellerman T, Reddy T, Harries A, et al. Randomized pharmacokinetic evaluation of different rifabutin doses in African HIV- infected tuberculosis patients on lopinavir/ritonavir-based antiretroviral therapy. BMC Pharmacol Toxicol. 2014;15:61.

47. Lan NT, Thu NT, Barrail-Tran A, Duc NH, Lan NN, Laureillard D, et al. Randomised pharmacokinetic trial of rifabutin with lopinavir/ritonavir-antiretroviral therapy in patients with HIV-associated tuberculosis in Vietnam. PLoS One. 2014;9(1):e84866.

48. Jenny-Avital ER, Joseph K. Rifamycin-resistant Mycobacterium tuberculosis in the highly active antiretroviral therapy era: a report of 3 relapses with acquired rifampin resistance following alternate-day rifabutin and boosted protease inhibitor therapy. Clin Infect Dis. 2009;48(10):1471–4.

49. Meintjes G, Wilkinson RJ, Morroni C, Pepper DJ, Rebe K, Rangaka MX, et al. Randomized placebo-controlled trial of prednisone for paradoxical tuberculosis-associated immune reconstitution inflammatory syndrome. AIDS. 2010;24(15):2381–90.

50. Dodd PJ, Gardiner E, Coghlan R, Seddon JA. Burden of childhood tuberculosis in 22 high-burden countries: a mathematical modelling study. Lancet Glob Health. 2014;2(8):E453–9.

51. Hesseling AC, Cotton MF, Jennings T, Whitelaw A, Johnson LF, Eley B, et al. High incidence of tuberculosis among HIV-infected infants: evidence from a south African population-based study highlights the need for improved tuberculosis control strategies. Clin Infect Dis. 2009;48(1):108–14.

52. Menzies HJ, Winston CA, Holtz TH, Cain KP, Mac Kenzie WR. Epidemiology of tuberculosis among US- and foreign-born children and adolescents in the United States, 1994–2007. Am J Public Health. 2010;100(9):1724–9.

53. CDC. Reported tuberculosis in the United States. Atlanta: US Department of health and Human Services, CDC; 2011.

54. Winston CA, Menzies HJ. Pediatric and adolescent tuberculosis in the United States, 2008–2010. Pediatrics. 2012;130(6):e1425–32.

55. Marais BJ, Gie RP, Schaaf HS, Hesseling AC, Obihara CC, Starke JJ, et al. The natural history of childhood intra-thoracic tuberculosis: a critical review of literature from the pre-chemotherapy era. Int J Tuberc Lung Dis. 2004;8(4):392–402.

56. CDC. Centers for disease control and prevention: guidelines for preventing the transmission of mycobacterium tuberculosis in health-care facilities, 1994. MMWR Morb Mortal Wkly Rep. 1994;44(RR-13):1–132.

57. Starke J. Transmission of mycobacterium tuberculosis to and from children and adolescents. Semin Pediatr Infect Dis. 2001;12(2):115–23.

58. Wallgren A. On the contagiousness of childhood tuberculosis. Acta Paediatr Scan. 1937;22:229–34.

59. Daly JF, Brown DS, Lincoln EM, Wilking VN. Endobronchial tuberculosis in children. Dis Chest. 1952;22(4):380–98.
60. Schaaf HS, Gie RP, Beyers N, Smuts N, Donald PR. Tuberculosis in infants less-than 3 months of age. Arch Dis Child. 1993;69(3): 371–4.
61. Miller FJW, Cashman JM. The natural history of peripheral tuberculous lymphadenitis associated with a visible primary focus. Lancet. 1955;268(6878):1286–9.
62. Seth V, Kabra SK, Jain Y, Semwal OP, Mukhopadhyaya S, Jensen RL. Tubercular lymphadenitis: clinical manifestations. Indian J Pediatr. 1995;62:565–70.
63. Marais BJ, Wright CA, Schaaf HS, Gie RP, Hesseling AC, Enarson DA, et al. Tuberculous lymphadenitis as a cause of persistent cervical lymphadenopathy in children from a tuberculosis-endemic area. Pediatr Infect Dis J. 2006;25(2):142–6.
64. Lincoln EM, Sordillo SVR, Davies PA. Tuberculous meningitis in children. J Pediatr. 1960;57:807–23.
65. Chiang SS, Khan FA, Milstein MB, Tolman AW, Benedetti A, Starke JR, et al. Treatment outcomes of childhood tuberculous meningitis: a systematic review and meta-analysis. Lancet Infect Dis. 2014;14(10):947–57.
66. Starke JR. Tuberculosis. An old disease but a new threat to the mother, fetus, and neonate. Clin Perinatol. 1997;24(1): 107–27.
67. Cantwell MF, Shehab ZM, Costello AM, Sands L, Green WF, Ewing Jr EP, et al. Brief report: congenital tuberculosis. N Engl J Med. 1994;330(15):1051–4.
68. Oberhelman RA, Soto-Castellares G, Gilman RH, Caviedes L, Castillo ME, Kolevic L, et al. Diagnostic approaches for paediatric tuberculosis by use of different specimen types, culture methods, and PCR: a prospective case–control study. Lancet Infect Dis. 2010;10(9):612–20.
69. Stockdale AJ, Duke T, Graham S, Kelly J. Evidence behind the WHO guidelines: hospital care for children: what is the diagnostic accuracy of gastric aspiration for the diagnosis of tuberculosis in children? J Trop Pediatr. 2010;56(5):291–8.
70. Nicol MP, Workman L, Isaacs W, Munro J, Black F, Eley B, et al. Accuracy of the Xpert MTB/RIF test for the diagnosis of pulmonary tuberculosis in children admitted to hospital in Cape Town, South Africa: a descriptive study. Lancet Infect Dis. 2011;11(11): 819–24.
71. Mukherjee A, Singh S, Lodha R, Singh V, Hesseling AC, Grewal HMS, et al. Ambulatory gastric lavages provide better yields of

mycobacterium tuberculosis than induced sputum in children with intrathoracic tuberculosis. Pediatr Infect Dis J. 2013;32(12):1313–7.

72. Jain SK, Ordonez A, Kinikar A, Gupte N, Thakar M, Mave V, et al. Pediatric tuberculosis in young children in India: a prospective study. Biomed Res Int. 2013;2013:783698.

73. Al-Aghbari N, Al-Sonboli N, Yassin MA, Coulter JB, Atef Z, Al-Eryani A, et al. Multiple sampling in one day to optimize smear microscopy in children with tuberculosis in Yemen. PLoS One. 2009;4(4):e5140.

74. Hatherill M, Hawkridge T, Zar HJ, Whitelaw A, Tameris M, Workman L, et al. Induced sputum or gastric lavage for community-based diagnosis of childhood pulmonary tuberculosis? Arch Dis Child. 2009;94(3):195–201.

75. Zar HJ, Hanslo D, Apolles P, Swingler G, Hussey G. Induced sputum versus gastric lavage for microbiological confirmation of pulmonary tuberculosis in infants and young children: a prospective study. Lancet. 2005;365(9454):130–4.

76. Salazar-Austin N, Ordonez A, Hsu A, Benson J, Mahesh M, Menachery E, et al. Extensively drug-resistant tuberculosis in a young child after travel to India. Lancet Infect Dis. 2015;15(12):1485–91.

77. Bates M, O'Grady J, Maeurer M, Tembo J, Chilukutu L, Chabala C, et al. Assessment of the Xpert MTB/RIF assay for diagnosis of tuberculosis with gastric lavage aspirates in children in sub-Saharan Africa: a prospective descriptive study. Lancet Infect Dis. 2013;13(1):36–42.

78. Zar HJ, Workman L, Isaacs W, Munro J, Black F, Eley B, et al. Rapid molecular diagnosis of pulmonary tuberculosis in children using nasopharyngeal specimens. Clin Infect Dis. 2012;55(8):1088–95.

79. Moore HA, Apolles P, de Villiers PJ, Zar HJ. Sputum induction for microbiological diagnosis of childhood pulmonary tuberculosis in a community setting. Int J Tuberc Lung Dis. 2011;15(9):1185–90. i.

80. Planting NS, Visser GL, Nicol MP, Workman L, Isaacs W, Zar HJ. Safety and efficacy of induced sputum in young children hospitalised with suspected pulmonary tuberculosis. Int J Tuberc Lung Dis. 2014;18(1):8–12.

81. Zar HJ, Workman L, Isaacs W, Dheda K, Zemanay W, Nicol MP. Rapid diagnosis of pulmonary tuberculosis in African children in a primary care setting by use of Xpert MTB/RIF on respiratory specimens: a prospective study. Lancet Glob Health. 2013;1(2):E97–104.

82. Swingler G, du Toit G, Andronikou S, van der Merwe L, Zar H. Diagnostic accuracy of chest radiography in detecting mediastinal

lymphadenopathy in suspected pulmonary tuberculosis. Arch Dis Child. 2005;90(11):1153–6.

83. Nicol MP, Spiers K, Workman L, Isaacs W, Munro J, Black F, et al. Xpert MTB/RIF testing of stool samples for the diagnosis of pulmonary tuberculosis in children. Clin Infect Dis. 2013;57(3):e18–21.

84. Nicol MP, Allen V, Workman L, Isaacs W, Munro J, Pienaar S, et al. Urine lipoarabinomannan testing for diagnosis of pulmonary tuberculosis in children: a prospective study. Lancet Glob Health. 2014;2(5):e278–84.

85. Kim W, Choi J, Cheon J, Kim I, Yeon K, Lee H. Pulmonary tuberculosis in infants: radiographic and CT findings. AJR Am J Roentgenol. 2006;187(4):1024–33.

86. Kaguthi G, Nduba V, Nyokabi J, Onchiri F, Gie R, Borgdorff M. Chest radiographs for pediatric TB diagnosis: interrater agreement and utility. Interdiscip Perspect Infect Dis. 2014;2014: 291841.

87. Mahesh M. Advances in CT technology and application to pediatric imaging. Pediatr Radiol. 2011;41 Suppl 2:493–7.

88. WHO. Guidance for national tuberculosis programmes on the management of tuberculosis in children. Geneva: World Health Organization; 2014.

89. ATS. American Thoracic Society/centers for disease control and prevention/infectious diseases society of America: treatment of tuberculosis. Am J Respir Crit Care Med. 2003;167:603–62.

90. McIlleron H, Willemse M, Werely CJ, Hussey GD, Schaaf HS, Smith PJ, et al. Isoniazid plasma concentrations in a cohort of South African children with tuberculosis: implications for international pediatric dosing guidelines. Clin Infect Dis. 2009;48(11):1547–53.

91. Graham SM, Bell DJ, Nyirongo S, Hartkoorn R, Ward SA, Molyneux EM. Low levels of pyrazinamide and ethambutol in children with tuberculosis and impact of age, nutritional status, and human immunodeficiency virus infection. Antimicrob Agents Chemother. 2006;50(2):407–13.

92. Thee S, Seddon JA, Donald PR, Seifart HI, Werely CJ, Hesseling AC, et al. Pharmacokinetics of isoniazid, rifampin, and pyrazinamide in children younger than two years of age with tuberculosis: evidence for implementation of revised world health organization recommendations. Antimicrob Agents Chemother. 2011;55(12):5560–7.

93. World Health Organization. Rapid Advice Treatment of tuberculosis in children. World Health Organization, Geneva; 2010.

http://apps.who.int/iris/bitstream/10665/44444/1/9789241500449_
eng.pdf. Last accessed March 11, 2016.

94. WHO. Ethambutol efficacy and toxicity: literature review and recommendations for daily and intermittent dosage in children. 2006.

95. Peloquin CA, Durbin D, Childs J, Sterling TR, Weiner M. Stability of antituberculosis drugs mixed in food. Clin Infect Dis. 2007;45(4):521.

96. Nachman S, Ahmed A, Amanullah F, Becerra MC, Botgros R, Brigden G, et al. Towards early inclusion of children in tuberculosis drugs trials: a consensus statement. Lancet Infect Dis. 2015;15(6):711–20.

97. Rodrigues LC, Diwan VK, Wheeler JG. Protective effect of BCG against tuberculous meningitis and miliary tuberculosis: a meta-analysis. Int J Epidemiol. 1993;22(6):1154–8.

98. Talbot EA, Perkins MD, Fagundes S, Silva M, Frothingham R. Disseminated bacille calmette-guerin disease after vaccination: case report and review. Clin Infect Dis. 1997;24(6):1139–46.

99. Hesseling AC, Marais BJ, Gie RP, Schaaf HS, Fine PEM, Godfrey-Faussett P, et al. The risk of disseminated Bacille Calmette-Guerin (BCG) disease in HIV-infected children. Vaccine. 2007;25(1):14–8.

100. Kruk A, Gie RP, Schaaf HS, Marais BJ. Symptom-based screening of child tuberculosis contacts: improved feasibility in resource-limited settings. Pediatrics. 2008;121(6):e1646–52.

101. Triasih R, Robertson CF, Duke T, Graham SM. A prospective evaluation of the symptom-based screening approach to the management of children who Are contacts of tuberculosis cases. Clin Infect Dis. 2015;60(1):12–8.

102. Saiman L, Colson P, Collaborative PT. Targeted tuberculin skin testing and treatment of latent tuberculosis infection in children and adolescents. Pediatrics. 2004;114(4):1175–201.

103. American Academy of Pediatrics [Tuberculosis]. In: Pickering LK, Baker CJ, Kimberlin DW, Long SS, eds. Red Book: 2015 Report of the Committee on Infectious Diseases. American Academy of Pediatrics, Elk Grove Village, IL; 2015:805–31.

104. Cohn DL, O'Brien RJ, Geiter LJ, Gordin FM, Hershfield E, Horsburgh CR, et al. Supplement – American Thoracic Society Centers for Disease Control and Prevention – Targeted tuberculin testing and treatment of latent tuberculosis infection. Am J Respir Crit Care Med. 2000;161(4):S221–47.

105. Markowitz N, Hansen NI, Wilcosky TC, Hopewell PC, Glassroth J, Kvale PA, et al. Tuberculin and anergy testing in

HIV-seropositive and HIV-seronegative persons. Pulmonary complications of HIV infection study group. Ann Intern Med. 1993;119(3):185–93.

106. Lincoln EM, Vera Cruz PG. Progress in treatment of tuberculosis. Results of antimicrobial therapy in a group of 420 children with tuberculosis. Pediatrics. 1960;25:1035–42.

107. Ferebee S, Mount FW, Anastasiades A. Prophylactic effects of isoniazid on primary tuberculosis in children; a preliminary report. Am Rev Tuberc. 1957;76(6):942–63.

108. Hsu KHK. Thirty years after isoniazid: its impact on tuberculosis in children and adolescents. JAMA. 1984;251(10):1283–5.

109. Villarino ME, Scott NA, Weis SE, Weiner M, Conde MB, Jones B, et al. Treatment for preventing tuberculosis in children and adolescents a randomized clinical trial of a 3-month, 12-dose regimen of a combination of rifapentine and isoniazid. JAMA Pediatr. 2015;169(3):247–55.

110. Spyridis NP, Spyridis PG, Gelesme A, Sypsa V, Valianatou M, Metsou F, et al. The effectiveness of a 9-month regimen of isoniazid alone versus 3- and 4-month regimens of isoniazid plus rifampin for treatment of latent tuberculosis infection in children: results of an 11-year randomized study. Clin Infect Dis. 2007;45(6):715–22.

111. van Zyl S, Marais BJ, Hesseling AC, Gie RP, Beyers N, Schaaf HS. Adherence to anti-tuberculosis chemoprophylaxis and treatment in children. Int J Tuberc Lung Dis. 2006;10(1):13–8.

112. Smieja MJ, Marchetti CA, Cook DJ, Smaill FM. Isoniazid for preventing tuberculosis in non-HIV infected persons. Cochrane Database Syst Rev. 2000;(2):CD001363.

113. International Union Against Tuberculosis Committee on Prophylaxis. Efficacy of various durations of isoniazid preventive therapy for tuberculosis: five years of follow-up in the IUAT trial. Bull World Health Organ. 1982;60(4):555–64.

114. Chang SH, Nahid P, Eitzman SR. Hepatotoxicity in children receiving isoniazid therapy for latent tuberculosis infection. J Pediatr Infect Dis Soc. 2007;3(3):221–7.

115. Donald PR. Antituberculous drug-induced hepatotoxicity in children. Pediat Rep. 2011;3:e16.

116. Cruz AT, Ahmed A, Mandalakas AM, Starke JR. Treatment of latent tuberculosis infection in children. J Pediatr Infect Dis Soc. 2013;27(10):913–9.

117. Weiner M, Savid R, Kenzie W, et al. Rifapentine Pharmacokinetics and Tolerabilty in Children and Adults Treated Once Weekly

With Rifapentine and Isoniazid for Latent Tuberculosis Infection. J Ped Infect Dis Soc 2014;3:132–45.

118. Cobelens F, van Deutekom H, Draayer-Jansen I, Schepp-Beelen A, van Gerven P, van Kessel R, et al. Risk of infection with Mycobacterium tuberculosis in travellers to areas of high tuberculosis endemicity. Lancet. 2000;356:461–5.

119. Andrews JR, Gandhi NR, Moodley P, Shah NS, Bohlken L, Moll AP, et al. Exogenous reinfection as a cause of multidrug-resistant and extensively drug-resistant tuberculosis in rural South Africa. J Infect Dis. World Health Organization, Geneva; 2008;198:1582–9.

120. Calver AD, Falmer AA, Murray M, Strauss OJ, Streicher EM, Hanekom M, et al. Emergence of increased resistance and extensively drug-resistant tuberculosis despite treatment adherence. South Africa Emerg Infect Dis. 2010;16(2):264–71.

121. Becerra MC, Appleton SC, Franke MF, Chalco K, Arteaga F, Bayona J, et al. Tuberculosis burden in households of patients with multidrug-resistant and extensively drug-resistant tuberculosis: a retrospective cohort study. Lancet. 2011;377(9760): 147–52.

122. Mitchison DA. How drug resistance merges as a result of poor compliance during short course chemotherapy for tuberculosis. Int J Tuberc Lung Dis. 1998;2(1):10–5.

123. Pasipanodya JG, McIlleron H, Burger A, Wash PA, Smith P, Gumbo T. Serum drug concentrations predictive of pulmonary tuberculosis outcomes. J Infect Dis. 2013;208(9):1464–73.

124. Srivastava S, Pasipanodya JG, Meek C, Leff R, Gumbo T. Multidrug-resistant tuberculosis not due to noncompliance but to between-patient pharmacokinetic variability. J Infect Dis. 2011;204:1951–9.

125. Dharmadhikari AS, Mphahlele M, Venter K, Stoltz A, Mathebula R, Masotla T, et al. Rapid impact of effect treatment on transmission of multidrug-resistant tuberculosis. Int J Tuberc Lung Dis. 2014;18(9):1019–25.

126. Bottger EC. The ins and outs of Mycobacterium tuberculosis drug susceptibility testing. Clin Microbiol Infect. 2011;17(8):1128–34.

127. Nuermberger E, Grosset J. Pharmacokinetic and pharmacodynamic issues in the treatment of mycobacterial infections. Eur J Clin Microbiol Infect Dis. 2004;23(4):243–55.

128. Lee J, Armstrong DT, Ssengooba W, Park JA, Yu Y, Mumbowa F, et al. Sensititre MYCOTB MIC plate for testing Mycobacterium tuberculosis susceptibility to first- and second-line drugs. Antimicrob Agents Chemother. 2014;58(1):11–8.

129. Hall L, Jude KP, Clark SL, Dionne K, Merson R, Boyer A, et al. Evaluation of the Sensititre MycoTB plate for susceptibility testing of the Mycobacterium tuberculosis complex against first- and second-line agents. J Clin Microbiol. 2012;50(11): 3732–4.

130. Zhang Y, Permar S, Sun ZH. Conditions that may affect the results of susceptibility testing of Mycobacterium tuberculosis to pyrazinamide. J Med Microbiol. 2002;51(1):42–9.

131. McDermott W, Tompsett R. Activation of pyrazinamide and nicotinamide in acidic environments in vitro. Am Rev Tuberc. 1954;70(4):748–54.

132. Scorpio A, Zhang Y. Mutations in pncA, a gene encoding pyrazinamidase/nicotinamidase, cause resistance to the antituberculous drug pyrazinamide in tubercle bacillus. Nat Med. 1996;2(6):662–7.

133. Boehme CC, Nabeta P, Hillemann D, Nicol MP, Shenai S, Krapp F, et al. Rapid molecular detection of tuberculosis and rifampin resistance. N Engl J Med. 2010;363(11):1005–15.

134. World Health Organization. Automated Real-Time Nucleic Acid Amplification Technology For Rapid And Simultaneous Detection Of Tuberculosis And Rifampicin Resistance: Xpert MTB/RIF System Policy Statement. World Health Organization, Geneva; 2011. http://apps.who.int/iris/bitstream/10665/ 44586/1/9789241501545_eng.pdf. Last accessed March 11, 2016.

135. Sanchez-Padilla E, Merker M, Beckert P, Jochims F, Dlamini T, Kahn P, et al. Detection of drug-resistant tuberculosis by Xpert MTB/RIF in Swaziland. N Engl J Med. 2015;372(12):1181–2.

136. Cepheid (2014). Cepheid, FIND & Rutgers Announce Collaboration for Next-Generation Innovations to Game-changing Xpert MTB/RIF Test [Press release]. Retrieved from http://ir.cepheid.com/releasedetail.cfm?releaseid=878540

137. Kempker RR, Vashakidze S, Solomonia N, Dzidzikashvili N, Blumberg HM. Surgical treatment of drug-resistant tuberculosis. Lancet Infect Dis. 2012;12(2):157–66.

138. World Health Organization. WHO treatment guidelines for drug-resistant tuberculosis 2016 Update. 2016. http://www.who. int/tb/MDRTBguidelines2016.pdf.

139. Cox H, Ford N. Linezolid for the treatment of complicated drug-resistant tuberculosis: a systematic review and meta-analysis. Int J Tuberc Lung Dis. 2012;16(4):447–54.

140. Gopal M, Padayatchi N, Metcalfe JZ, O'Donnell MR. Systematic review of clofazimine for the treatment of drug-resistant tuberculosis. Int J Tuberc Lung Dis. 2013;17(8):1001–7.

141. WHO. The use of bedaquiline in the treatment of multidrug resistant tuberculosis. Geneva: WHO; 2013.
142. WHO. The use of delamanid in the treatment of multidrug-resistant tuberculosis interim policy guidance. Geneva: WHO; 2014.
143. Gillespie SH, Crook AM, McHugh TD, Mendel CM, Meredith SK, Murray SR, et al. Four-month moxifloxacin-based regimens for drug-sensitive tuberculosis. N Engl J Med. 2014; 371(17):1577–87.
144. Jindani A, Harrison TS, Nunn AJ, Phillips PP, Churchyard GJ, Charalambous S, et al. High-dose rifapentine with moxifloxacin for pulmonary tuberculosis. N Engl J Med. 2014;371(17): 1599–608.
145. Falzon D, Jaramillo E, Schunemann HJ, Arentz M, Bauer M, Bayona J, et al. WHO guidelines for the programmatic management of drug-resistant tuberculosis: 2011 update. Eur Respir J. 2011;38(3):516–28.
146. Aung K, Van Deun A, Declercq E, Sarker M, Das P, Hossain M, et al. Successful '9-month Bangladesh regimen' for multidrug-resistant tuberculosis among over 500 consecutive patients. Int J Tuberc Lung Dis. 2014;18:1180–7.
147. Piubello A, Harouna S, Souleymane M, Boukary I, Morou S, Daouda M, et al. High cure rate with standardised short-course multidrug-resistant tuberculosis treatment in Niger: no relapses. Int J Tuberc Lung Dis. 2014;18:1188–94.
148. Nathanson E, Lambregts-van Weezenbeek C, Rich ML, Gupta R, Bayona J, Blöndal K, et al. Multi-drug resistant tuberculosis management in resource-limited settings. Emerg Infect Dis. 2006;12(9):1389–97.
149. Orenstein EW, Basu S, Shah NS, Andrews JR, Friedland GH, Moll AP, et al. Treatment outcomes among patients with multidrug-resistant tuberculosis: systematic review and meta-analysis. Lancet Infect Dis. 2009;9:153–61.
150. Johnston JC, Shahidi NC, Sadatsafavi M, Fitzgerald JM. Treatment outcomes of multidrug-resistant tuberculosis: a systematic review and meta-analysis. PLoS One. 2009;4(9):e6914.
151. Ahuja SD, Ashkin D, Avendano M, Banerjee R, Bauer M, Bayona JN, et al. Multidrug resistant pulmonary tuberculosis treatment regimens and patient outcomes: an individual patient data meta-analysis of 9,153 patients. PLoS Med. 2012;9(8): e1001300.
152. Gandhi NR, Moll AP, Sturm AW, Pawinski R, Govender T, Lalloo U, et al. Extensively drug-resistant tuberculosis as a

cause of death in patients co-infected with tuberculosis and HIV in a rural area of South Africa. Lancet. 2006;368:1575–80.

153. Jacobson KR, Tierney DB, Jeon CY, Mitnick CD, Murray MB. Treatment outcomes among patients with extensively drug-resistant tuberculosis: systematic review and meta-analysis. Clinical Infect Dis. 2010;51(1):6–14.

154. Pietersen E, Ignatius E, Streicher EM, Mastrapa B, Padanilam X, Pooran A, et al. Long-term outcomes of patients with extensively drug-resistant tuberculosis in South Africa: a cohort study. Lancet. 2014;383(9924):1230–9.

155. Kwon YS, Kim YH, Suh GY, Chung MP, Kim H, Kwon OJ, et al. Treatment outcomes for HIV-uninfected patients with multidrug-resistant and extensively drug-resistant tuberculosis. Clinical Infect Dis. 2008;47:496–502.

156. Keshavjee S, Gelmanova IY, Farmer PE, Mishustin SP, Strelis AK, Andreev YG, et al. Treatment of extensively drug-resistant tuberculosis in Tomsk, Russia: a retrospective cohort study. Lancet. 2008;372(9647):1403–9.

157. Banerjee R, Allen J, Westenhouse J, Oh P, Elms W, Desmond E, et al. Extensively drug-resistant tuberculosis in california, 1993–2006. Clin Infect Dis. 2008;47(4):450–7.

158. Mitnick CD, Shin SS, Seung KJ, Rich ML, Atwood SS, Furin JJ, et al. Comprehensive treatment of extensively drug-resistant tuberculosis. N Engl J Med. 2008;359(6):563–74.

159. Jeon DS, Kim DH, Kang HS, Hwang SH, Min JH, Kim JH, et al. Survival and predictors of outcomes in non-HIV-infected patients with extensively drug-resistant tuberculosis. Int J Tuberc Lung Dis. 2009;13(5):594–600.

160. Seddon JA, Hesseling AC, Finlayson H, Fielding K, Cox H, Hughes J, et al. Preventive therapy for child contacts of multidrug-resistant tuberculosis: a prospective cohort study. Clin Infect Dis. 2013;57(12):1676–84.

161. Bamrah S, Brostrom R, Dorina F, Setik L, Song R, Kawamura LM, et al. Treatment for LTBI in contacts of MDR-TB patients, Federated States of Micronesia, 2009–2012. Int J Tuberc Lung Dis. 2014;18(8):912–8.

Chapter 7
Emerging Therapies

Gyanu Lamichhane and Jacques H. Grosset

7.1 Introduction

Despite the tremendous efficacy of the treatment of tuberculosis (TB) which can cure the disease in 6 months and resulted in the dramatic reduction of patient sufferings from TB, the success of TB treatment has been hampered by the development of resistance to existing drugs in numerous parts of the world [1]. This, in turn, has reactivated research on drugs active against TB (Table 7.1), on vaccines safer and more efficacious than BCG, and on host-directed therapies. The current chapter is providing a summary of the state of the art in these fields [2].

G. Lamichhane
Department of Medicine, Johns Hopkins University,
Orleans St 1550, Baltimore, MD 21287, USA
e-mail: lamichhane@jhu.edu

J.H. Grosset (✉)
Department of Medicine, Johns Hopkins University School of Medicine, 1550 Orleans St, Rm 105, Baltimore, MD 21231, USA
e-mail: jgrosse4@jhmi.edu

J.H. Grosset, R.E. Chaisson (eds.), *Handbook of Tuberculosis*,   191
DOI 10.1007/978-3-319-26273-4_7,
© Springer International Publishing Switzerland 2017

TABLE 7.1 Newly understudy antimicrobial drugs for tuberculosis

Drugs	Brand name	References
Drugs in preclinical development		
Q203	Imidazopyridine amide	[3, 4]
Benzothiazinones	BTZ043	[5]
	PBTZ169	[6]
New registered anti-TB drugs		
Diarylquinoline	TMC, bedaquiline (Sirturo)	[4, 7–24]
Nitro-dihydro-imidazo-oxazoles	Delamanid (Deltyba)	[25–28]
	Pretomanid (PA-824)	[29–33]
	TBA-354	[34–36]
Drugs repurposed for their anti-TB activity		
Oxazolidinones	Linezolid (Zyvox)	[37–48]
	Sutezolid (PNU100480)	[37, 38, 40, 41, 49–52]
	Tedizolid (Sivextro)	[53–56]
Fluoroquinolones	Levofloxacin (Levaquin)	[57]
	Moxifloxacin (Avelox)	[58–68]
β-Lactams	Carbapenems	[69–80]
Existing TB drugs on reevaluation		
Rifapentine	Priftin	[81, 82]
Clofazimine	Lamprene, B663	[83–92]

7.2   The Drugs in Preclinical Development

7.2.1   Q203

Q203 is an imidazopyridine amide that blocks *Mycobacterium tuberculosis* (*M.tb*) growth by targeting the respiratory cytochrome bc_1 complex (ubiquinol: cytochrome *c* oxidoreductase), like clofazimine [3]. As the bc_1 complex is the first step in the electron transfer chain, the action of Q203 results in rapid depletion of intracellular ATP, a property in common with bedaquiline [4]. Q203 inhibits the growth of drug-susceptible and drug-resistant clinical isolates of *M.tb* in broth medium at the low nanomolar range (2.7nM) and was active in a mouse model of TB at a dose less than 1 mg per kg body weight. In addition, Q203 displays pharmacokinetic and safety profiles compatible with once-daily dosing. Together, these data suggest that Q203 is a promising new clinical candidate for TB treatment.

7.2.2   Benzothiazinones

Benzothiazinones (BTZ) are novel class of antimycobacterials that act by blocking the synthesis of decaprenyl-phospho-arabinose, the precursor of the arabinans in the mycobacterial cell wall [5]. The lead compound BTZ043 has an MIC of 0.001 µg/ml for *M.tb* and demonstrated to be fully compatible with all the other approved or experimental TB drugs tested. Both BTZ043 and the 2-piperazino-benzothiazinone 169 (PBTZ169), a new preclinical drug candidate, act synergistically in vitro with bedaquiline, an ATP synthase inhibitor [6]. Compared to BTZ043, PBTZ169 has improved potency, safety, and efficacy in zebra fish and mouse models of TB, and highly encouraging results were obtained against chronic murine TB when PBTZ169 was administered in combination with bedaquiline and/or pyrazinamide.

7.3   The Newly Registered Anti-Tuberculosis Drugs and Related Molecules

7.3.1   The Diarylquinoline, Bedaquiline (TMC 207)

Under the brand name of Sirturo™, the diarylquinoline (bedaquiline) has been granted regulatory approval under accelerated or conditional procedures by the US Food and Drug Administration (USFDA) in December 2012 [7, 8] and conditional approval by the European Medicines Agency (EMA) in February 2014 [9]. As an interim recommendation, a WHO Expert Group [10] suggested that bedaquiline may be added to the WHO-recommended regimen for multidrug-resistant (MDR) TB adult patients when an effective treatment regimen containing four second-line drugs in addition to pyrazinamide, according to WHO recommendations, cannot be designed and when there is documented evidence of resistance to any fluoroquinolone in addition to MDR.

Bedaquiline belongs to a new chemical family that targets the proton pump of adenosine triphosphate (ATP) synthase and leads to inadequate synthesis of ATP. Bedaquiline has an MIC for *M.tb* of 0.06 µg/ml, no cross-resistance with existing anti-TB, and a time-dependent activity driven by the time over MIC [4]. At concentrations 10 times the MIC and even 100 times the MIC in 7H9 broth, the drug was highly bactericidal against *M.tb*, but this was only observed after 6 days of incubation and not earlier, indicating that the drug has no early bactericidal activity and needs to accumulate to express its antimicrobial activity.

In mice, after a single dose of 30 mg/kg of bedaquiline, the C_{max} reached 2.14 µg/ml within 3 h. The drug is metabolized primarily by the cytochrome P_{450} 3A4 (CYP3A4) into its major *N*-mono-desmethyl metabolite which is about 5 times less active than the parent compound. Both compounds are eliminated with long terminal half-lives of 50–60 h in mice, suggesting considerable tissue binding. The numerous studies that where conducted in the mouse model of TB [4, 11–17] have shown that bedaquiline has an impressive anti-TB activity when given alone or in combination with other drugs, especially pyrazinamide. However, it should be noted that absence of pyrazinamide or a rifamycin in any bedaquiline-containing regimen resulted a significant decrease in sterilizing activity [11, 17].

In humans, the C_{max} reached 1.2 ± 0.39 µg/ml within 4 h after an oral dose of 100 mg and 5.5 ± 2.96 µg/ml within 4 h after a dose of 400 mg [18]. The half-life is estimated to be ≥ 24 h, suggesting also considerable tissue binding of bedaquiline in humans. The steady-state plasma concentration is on average close to 1.0 µg/ml.

Up to now, seven clinical studies have been performed with bedaquiline, three studies of the early bactericidal activity (EBA) of bedaquiline in patients with drug-susceptible TB, and four studies of the activity of bedaquiline in the treatment of patients with multidrug-resistant tuberculosis.

The first EBA study was of 7 days' duration and demonstrated that bedaquiline had delayed and dose-dependent bactericidal activity and was not inducing serious side effects [18]. The second EBA study [19] compared the activity for 14 days of bedaquiline alone or in combination with pyrazinamide or pretomanid (PA-824) with the four-drug standard regimen for TB as control. It confirmed the lack of bactericidal activity of bedaquiline during the first 7 days despite the prescription of huge loading doses, the potent bactericidal activity of bedaquiline beyond the 7th day, and the synergism between bedaquiline and pyrazinamide. The third EBA study [20] mainly assessed the 14-day activity of four combined regimens of bedaquiline in permutations with pyrazinamide, pretomanid (PA-824), and clofazimine and the four-drug standard regimen for TB as control. None of the drug combinations with bedaquiline had bactericidal activity different from the control.

The first study of the activity of bedaquiline in the treatment of patients with multidrug-resistant TB was an 8-week randomized trial [21] involving a total of 47 patients treated with either a five-drug control regimen including kanamycin, ofloxacin, ethionamide, pyrazinamide, and cycloserine or the same drug regimen reinforced by bedaquiline at 400 mg daily for 2 weeks, followed by 200 mg three times a week for 6 weeks. The bedaquiline-containing regimen resulted in a much higher proportion of culture conversion by the end of 8 weeks, 48 % versus 9 % ($p = 0.003$).

The second study of treatment of multidrug-resistant TB with bedaquiline [22] was the 24-week (6-month) and 104-week (2-year) follow-up of the 47 patients involved in the previous study. The important information was the time to 50 % culture conversion: 78 days for patients with bedaquiline and 129 days for patients without bedaquiline.

The third study of treatment of multidrug-resistant TB with bedaquiline [23] involved 160 patients randomized to a preferred five-drug background regimen (usually ethionamide, pyrazinamide, ofloxacin, kanamycin, and cycloserine) with and without bedaquiline for 24 weeks followed for all patients by the background regimen for a further 96-week period (total 120 weeks). Bedaquiline was administered as 400 mg once daily for 2 weeks and then as 200 mg thrice weekly for 22 weeks. Faster culture conversion, 83 days versus 125 days ($p < 0.001$), and higher rate of culture conversion at 24 weeks, 58 % versus 79 % ($p = 0.008$), were observed among patients who had received bedaquiline. At the end of the study, at 120 weeks, the cure rate was 58 % among bedaquiline-treated patients and only 32 % in the other patients. There were, however, ten deaths in the bedaquiline group versus two in the other group, though no causal pattern was evident.

The fourth study of treatment of multidrug-resistant TB with bedaquiline [24] involved 35 patients who received compassionate bedaquiline combined with a median of 4 second-line drugs. At 6 months of bedaquiline treatment, culture conversion was achieved in 28 out of 29 (97 %) patients who were culture positive at the time of bedaquiline initiation. The median time to culture conversion was very similar to those observed in the previous Diacon studies [22, 23].

Although this most recent study involved the compassionate use of bedaquiline and was devoid of a control regimen without bedaquiline, it confirmed the potential of bedaquiline for the treatment of multidrug-resistant TB.

7.3.2   The Nitro-dihydro-imidazo-oxazoles

The nitro-dihydro-imidazo-oxazole class of compounds are derivatives of metronidazole that inhibit mycolic acid synthesis and have potent in vitro and in vivo activity against both drug-susceptible and drug-resistant strains of *M.tb*. Three derivatives are available, delamanid (OPC-67683) recommended as Deltyba by the European Medicines Agency for the treatment of multidrug-resistant forms of tuberculosis [9]; pretomanid (PA-824) that is evaluated in novel drug regimens for TB, including for drug-resistant TB patients; and TBA-354, a new nitro-imidazole derivative with potentially superior pharmacokinetic profile compared to delamanid and pretomanid.

7.3.3   Delamanid (OPC-67683, Deltyba)

Delamanid [25] is a nitromidazo-oxazole of which the MIC for *M.tb*, both susceptible and resistant to other drugs, is in the range of 0.006–0.012 µg/ml, about 10 times lower than the MIC of pretomanid (PA-824). Delamanid is potent against intracellular *M.tb*, where its activity at a concentration of 0.1 µg/ml was equivalent to that of RIF at a concentration of 1–3 µg/ml. In murine models, delamanid has limited bioavailability but long half-life: given at a dose of 2.5 mg/kg, the C_{max} was 0.29 µg/ml and half-life of 7.6 h. Combined with RIF and PZA, it caused more rapid culture conversion of lung tissue than the standard regimen of RIF + INH + PZA + EMB

In humans, delamanid is well tolerated at oral doses of 100, 200, 300, or 400 mg given daily for a 14-day extended EBA study. Its exposure is less than dosage proportional, reaches a plateau at 300 mg with a C_{max} of 0.352 µg/ml, and causes a decline in CFU counts of 0.9 $\log_{10}$ per ml of sputum over 14 days [26]. In the treatment of patients with multidrug-resistant TB, the rate of culture conversion at 2 months is of 29.6 % and 45.4 % in patients treated with an optimized background drug regimen without and with 100 to 200 mg twice daily of delamanid [27], respectively. The rate of favorable results at 24 months was 44 and 65 % among patients treated with delamanid [28] for less than 2 months (4/9) and for at least 6 months (11/17), respectively.

7.3.4   Pretomanid (PA-824)

Pretomanid [29] is a nitroimidazo-oxazine with an MIC of 0.125 µg/ml, ten times higher than that of delamanid, for both drug-susceptible and drug-resistant strains of *M.tb*. However, in humans, its C_{max} is about 10 times higher than the C_{max} of delamanid [30], and it is bactericidal against actively replicating as well as nonreplicating organisms.

In murine models of TB, PA-824 has bactericidal activity during both the initial and the continuation phases of treatment [31]. When dosed daily in combination with the fluoroquinolone, moxifloxacin, and pyrazinamide, it contributes an impressive sterilizing regimen [32] which has the potential to shorten the duration of treatment for drug-susceptible as well as drug-resistant TB because it contains no rifampin and no isoniazid. Such potential has been confirmed in an EBA study in humans [19] that demonstrated that the 3-drug combination, PA 824+ MXF + PZA, resulted at day 14 in 3 $\log_{10}$ CFU killing, significantly more than the 2$\log_{10}$ killing obtained with the standard 4-drug combination. The recent clinical evaluation of 8 weeks of treatment with the combination of PA-824, moxifloxacin, and pyrazinamide in patients with drug-sensitive and multidrug-resistant pulmonary TB confirms the previous EBA results [33].

7.3.5   TBA-354

TBA-354 is a next-generation derivative [34] that has in vitro potency superior to that of pretomanid and greater meta-bolic stability than delamanid. Its MIC for drug-susceptible and drug-resistant *M.tb* is 0.006 μg/ml compared to 0.125 μg/ml for pretomanid and 0.012 μg/ml for delamanid [35]. The pharmacokinetic and pharmacodynamic parameters were studied in mice [35, 36]: after oral doses of 2, 3, 30, and 100 mg/kg of TBA-354, the C_{max} was 1.78, 1.65, 9.26, and 12.8; the half-life was 15.6, 8.0, 11.0, and 12.0; and the $AUC_{0\text{-inf}}$ (μg.h/ml) was 35.3, 22.7, 153, and 242, respectively. TBA has longer plasma half-life and better AUC than PA-824. At 100 mg/kg in the mouse model of TB, TBA-354 is at least as potent as delamanid and more potent than pretomanid. Therefore, a phase 1 clinical trial was initiated. However, in January 2016, TB Alliance announced that it voluntarily halted further dosing of its phase 1 compound, TBA-354, due to unexpected signs detected in clinical trial participants who were administered the compound. The organization has now made a decision to end this clinical trial program.

7.4   Drugs Repurposed for Their Anti-Tuberculosis Activity

7.4.1   The Oxazolidinones

The oxazolidinones, which contain 2-oxazolidinone-fluorobenezene backbone, belong to a class of antibiotics directed at the inhibition of translation, the third stage of protein biosynthesis [37].

Linezolid

Linezolid released in 2000 by Upjohn is the first FDA-approved oxazolidinone for the treatment of nosocomial pneumonia and skin and soft tissue infections caused by Gram-positive bacteria [38]. The most common dosing regimen is 600 mg twice daily, the Cmax is 17.8 ± 6.03 μg/ml at steady state between 1 and 2 h after oral administration of this dosing regimen, and the half-life is 5–7 h [39]. Linezolid has been used off label against multidrug-resistant TB because its MIC50 for *M.tb* is 0.25 and its MIC90 is of 0.50 μg/ml [40]. It has been the object of a 7-day EBA study in which new patients with smear-positive pulmonary TB received either linezolid 600 mg twice or once daily or isoniazid 300 mg once daily as control [41]. The mean daily decline of sputum CFU counts was $0.16 \log_{10}$/ml for isoniazid, $0.04 \log_{10}$/ml for linezolid 600 mg twice a day, and $0.09 \log_{10}$/ml for linezolid 600 mg once a day, thus demonstrating a very limited early bactericidal activity of linezolid. Furthermore, its long-term administration required for the treatment of MDR TB patients is hampered by major side effects such as anemia, thrombocytopenia, and/or peripheral and optic neuropathy, related to the impairment of mitochondrial protein synthesis [42–44]. Among 38 patients with extensively drug-resistant tuberculosis who received linezolid 600 mg once a day added to their background regimen, 34 (87 %) were culture negative by 6 months and 27 (71 %) were culture negative by 12 months and remained culture negative 1 year after termination of the study [45, 46]. Clinically adverse events were observed in 82 % of patients and resistance to linezolid developed in 10 %. In a systematic review [47] reporting the outcome of treatment of 148 patients with linezolid, the pooled proportion of success was 68 % despite the high frequency of side effects that led to discontinuing linezolid in 36 % of treated patients. To limit the frequency and seriousness of side effects related to mitochondrial toxicity, thrice-weekly administration of linezolid 600 or 1200 mg has been successfully tried in an observational study of ten patients, suggesting that linezolid toxicity may be reduced by longer exposure to low levels of linezolid [48].

Sutezolid

Sutezolid (PNU100480 /PNU) is a linezolid analogue with similar MICs for *M.tb* (MIC_{50} of 0.25 and MIC_{90} of 0.50 µg/ml) [37, 40] which has been developed by Pfizer for better *in vivo* activity and hopefully less toxicity [37, 38]. It has received Orphan Drug designation in both USA and European Union. In the murine model, compared with linezolid alone, sutezolid at 25 mg/kg was as potent as linezolid at 100 mg/kg, and at 50 mg/kg was more potent than linezolid at 260 mg/kg [49]. Moreover, the addition of sutezolid improved the bactericidal activities of regimens containing any of the current first-line drugs [50].

The safety, tolerability, pharmacokinetics, and pharmacodynamics of sutezolid were assessed in healthy volunteers at doses of either 100, 300, or 600 mg twice daily or 1200 mg once daily for 14 days. A fifth group received sutezolid at 600 mg twice daily for 28 days to which pyrazinamide at 25 mg/kg was added on days 27 and 28. A sixth group was given linezolid at 300 mg daily for 4 days. All doses were safe and well tolerated [51]. In subjects receiving twice daily 600 mg of sutezolid, the $t_{1/2}$ was 2.9 h and the C_{max} was 0.94 µg/ml quite lower than the C_{max} of 17.8 ± 6.03 µg/ml obtained with similar dosing of linezolid, but trough concentrations were maintained at or above the MIC. Measured by the whole blood activity assay, the maximal bactericidal effect of sutezolid was displayed at 600 mg twice daily, and the bactericidal effect of linezolid at 300 mg once daily was significantly less. Finally a clinical trial [52] of 14-day duration was conducted among new sputum smear-positive TB patients treated with sutezolid 600 mg twice daily, 1200 mg once daily, or standard first-line drug regimen (RHZE). Actually there was limited bactericidal activity of sutezolid at the chosen doses (about 1.23 $\log_{10}$ CFU killing in 14 days) compared to that of the standard RHZE treatment (about 2.75 $\log_{10}$ CFU killing in 14 days). Furthermore, the microbial killing of sutezolid was similar for twice 600 mg and once 1200 mg and not different from that reported with linezolid at similar dosing [41].

Tedizolid

Tedizolid (Sivextro, tedizolid phosphate) is the second of the oxazolidinones to have been approved (on June 20, 2014) by the US Food and Drug Administration to treat adults with acute bacterial skin and skin structure infections. Tedizolid phosphate (TR-701) is a prodrug that is transformed in the serum into the active drug tedizolid (TR-700) that acts like other oxazolidinones by inhibiting protein synthesis. Against *M.tb*, tedizolid, like linezolid and sutezolid, has MIC_{50} and MIC_{90} of 0.25 and 0.5 µg/ml, respectively, against susceptible and multidrug-resistant isolates [53]. In its approved indication, tedizolid is administered once daily at 200 mg for 6 days and is available in intravenous and oral formulations with an estimated bioavailability of 91.47 %. A 200 mg oral dose results in a C_{max} of 1.8 µg/ml inferior to the C_{max} of 12–14 µg/ml of linezolid after 600 mg twice daily, but the half-life is 11 h, whereas the half-life of linezolid is 3–4 h after 600 mg twice daily [54]. Compared to linezolid, the peak of exposure to tedizolid is lower, for a dose three times lower, but the duration of exposure to tedizolid is longer. In a first randomized study of treatment of acute bacterial skin infections [55], once-daily oral tedizolid 200 mg for 6 days among 332 patients was statistically non-inferior to twice-daily oral linezolid 600 mg for 10 days among 335 patients. In a second similar randomized study [56], once-daily intravenous tedizolid 200 mg (332 patients) for 6 days was statistically non-inferior to twice-daily oral linezolid 600 mg (334 patients) for 10 days. Tedizolid may therefore be considered as active as linezolid at 1/6 of the daily dose or 1.3 of the unit dose against acute bacterial skin infections. While tedizolid has not been administered to patients for more than 6 days, its favorable PK profile including linearity, low accumulation over time, low free drug systemic exposure, and a clean 9-month neurotoxicity rat study at up to 8 times the human equivalent dose suggest that it may be safer than linezolid after prolonged administration. Because of such characteristics, the antimicrobial activity and safety profile of tedizolid are worth to be investigated in TB patients.

7.4.2 The Fluoroquinolones

Quinolones are synthetic compounds active on the microbial DNA gyrases, enzymes needed for DNA replication. The majority of quinolones in clinical use are fluoroquinolones, which contain a fluorine atom. Third-generation quinolones have increased in vitro activity against *M.tb* as well as augmented pharmacokinetic parameters that result in enhanced pharmacodynamic characteristics. Among fluoroquinolones, the most active against *M.tb* [57] are levofloxacin, the levo isomer of the racemate ofloxacin, gatifloxacin (now taken off the market because of side effects including dysglycemia), and moxifloxacin (MXF) which has an MIC90 of 0.5 μg/ml for *M.tb*. In humans, after an oral dose of 400 mg, the maximum serum concentration of MXF is 3.2–4.5 μg/ml and the half-life is 9–12 h [58].

Moxifloxacin has bactericidal activity similar to that of INH against multiplying *M.tb* both in the murine model of TB [59, 60] and in humans [61]. Even the substitution of 400 mg MXF for 300 mg INH in the standard drug regimen for pulmonary TB [62] resulted in a marginally ($p = 0.37$) higher proportion, 60.4 % versus 54.9 %, of 2-month sputum culture conversion to negative. For this reason, the incorporation of MXF in the first-line drug regimen for TB was thought to allow for shortening treatment duration. Actually several studies [63, 64] demonstrated that the substitution of MXF or gatifloxacin for ethambutol resulted in a significantly more rapid decline of sputum CFU counts during the first 2 months and a higher culture conversion rate at the 2-month time point. However, such improved bactericidal activity as measured by the culture conversion rate at the 2-month time point was translated into improved sterilizing activity as measured by the relapse rate after stopping treatment for 4 months neither in the OFLOTUB Trial [65] nor in the REMox TB Trial [66] nor in the RIFAQUIN Trial despite combination with intermittent 15 mg/kg dose of rifapentine in this trial [67]. It can be concluded that MXF like isoniazid has potent bactericidal activity against *M.tb* but limited sterilizing activity. Because of their excellent bactericidal activity, fluoroquinolones are the backbone of combined drug regimens for MDR-TB [68]. Because levofloxacin can be given at higher daily doses than MXF, a clinical trial named Opti-Q (ClinicalTrials.gov Identifier: NCT01918397) has been designed to assess its efficacy and safety and is currently in progress. MDR-TB patients are treated with an optimized background regimen (OBR) supplemented by four different daily doses of 11, 14, 17, and 20 mg/kg/day of levofloxacin.

7.4.3   The β-Lactams

Although β-lactams comprise over 50 % of antibiotics used globally to treat bacterial infections in humans [69, 70], this class of drugs is rarely considered for treatment of *M.tb* infection. It has been argued that chromosomally encoded β-lactamase of *M.tb* hydrolyzes β-lactams and therefore renders them ineffective against this pathogen [71]. While this is largely true for existing penicillins, cephalosporins, and monobactams, it was recently demonstrated that carbapenem class of β-lactams are poor substrates (or slow inhibitors) of *M.tb* β-lactamase [72]. This study also reported potent activity of meropenem and imipenem, alone and in combination with clavulanic acid, against drug-susceptible and drug-resistant *M.tb*.

β-lactams derive their activity by inhibiting biosynthesis of peptidoglycan, a layer that encapsulates the plasma membrane and is required for survival and growth of *M.tb*. The final step of peptidoglycan biosynthesis requires two enzymes, L,D-transpeptidases and D,D-transpeptidases (also known as penicillin-binding proteins), that generate 3–3 and 4–3 transpeptide bonds, thereby polymerizing the peptidoglycan monomers [73–75]. While penicillins, cephalosporins, and monobactams inhibit D,D-transpeptidases, carbapenems are unique as they inhibit both D,D- and L,D-transpeptidases. Hence, carbapenems are effective in inhibiting *M.tb* growth not only because they are poor substrates of *M.tb* β-lactamases [72], but primarily because they (and only they) bind to and inhibit L,D-transpeptidases.

Parenterally administered carbapenems such as meropenem, imipenem, and doripenem and orally bioavailable faropenem and tebipenem exhibit in vitro activity against drug-susceptible and drug-resistant strains of *M.tb* [72, 76–79]. In vitro potencies of carbapenems determined on the basis of minimum inhibitory concentration (MIC) rank as tebipenem > faropenem = biapenem = doripenem > meropenem > ertapenem > imipenem [76, 79]. Although a comprehensive clinical trial of activity of the carbapenems against *M.tb* infection in humans is pending, their use for successful treatment of extensively drug-resistant TB has been reported recently [80]. Clavulanic acid has been shown to modestly increase potency of some carbapenems in vitro [72, 79]. It is not known if this synergy will be maintained in humans. In addition, dehydropeptidase I found in the renal brush border cells are known to metabolize and inactivate carbapenems. Cilastatin has been used to protect carbapenems against this enzyme. As activity of carbapenems depends on time above MIC or effective exposure, any agent that can prolong half-life and bioavailability of these drugs will likely increase their utility to treat *M.tb* infection. In summary, based on emerging evidence, carbapenems represent a promising class of drugs for treatment of TB.

7.5   Existing Tuberculosis Drugs on Reevaluation

7.5.1   Rifapentine

Rifapentine is the 3-[(4-cyclopentyl-l-piperazinyl) iminomethyl] rifamycin SV derivative. Its MIC for *M.tb* is 0.06 μg/ml, while that of the most widely used rifamycin derivative, rifampicin, is 0.25 μg/ml. Rifapentine is more highly protein bound (97 %) than of rifampicin (85 %). As its half-life ($t_{1/2}$) is 10–15 h, i.e., five times longer than the 2–3 h $t_{1/2}$ of rifampicin, it was assumed that rifapentine would provide longer exposure of *M.tb* to active rifamycin and consequently would allow once-weekly treatment of TB in combination with isoniazid. In fact, such once-weekly drug combination in the continuation phase of tuberculosis treatment resulted in high rates of TB relapses in patients with cavitary TB and/or HIV positivity with rifamycin-mono-resistant bacilli. Moreover, once-weekly isoniazid-rifapentine was shown to be less active than thrice- or twice-weekly isoniazid-rifampicin. It has been suggested that the high protein binding of rifapentine was partially responsible for the suboptimal activity observed in once-weekly regimens.

Another possibility to improve the effectiveness of rifapentine is to increase the rhythm of rifapentine administration for augmenting drug exposure. In the mouse model of TB, five days/week administration of 10 mg/kg rifapentine-isoniazid and pyrazinamide for 3 months was curing mice and preventing any relapse, whereas the standard rifampicin-containing daily regimen required 6 months to prevent relapse in all mice. Building on the mouse data, Dorman et al conducted a phase 2 clinical trial and found 10 mg/kg of daily rifapentine to be as safe as, but not more efficacious than 10 mg/kg of daily rifampin during the first 8 weeks of combination TB chemotherapy. But a phase 1 clinical trial showed that rifapentine doses up to 20 mg/kg administered daily were well tolerated and safe in healthy volunteers [81]. Then, a dose-ranging (10, 15, and 20 mg/kg) clinical trial [82] was conducted to determine the optimal dose of daily rifapentine during the first 8 weeks (intensive phase) of combination treatment for pulmonary TB. It showed that the substitution of higher dose of rifapentine, 15 and 20 mg/kg, for rifampin improves the antimicrobial activity of combination chemotherapy. As high doses of rifapentine were safe and well tolerated, this clinical trial supports the evaluation of high-dose daily rifapentine containing regimens of less than 6-month duration in phase 3 clinical trials.

7.5.2   Clofazimine

Clofazimine, B663 or lamprene, is a fat-soluble rimino-phenazine dye developed by Barry et al. in the 1950s as an antituberculosis drug [83]. Despite quite favorable experimental findings, clofazimine was not considered for antituberculosis treatment, likely due to fears related to the red skin discoloration induced by the phenazine dye and to the success of the three-drug combination of streptomycin, isoniazid, and para-aminosalicylic acid in the treatment of TB at the time of clofazimine development. Because of its activity against *M. leprae* and its anti-inflammatory properties, clofazimine became a drug for leprosy. A short-lived renewal of interest in clofazimine for treatment of infections due to mycobacteria other than *M. leprae* was triggered by its apparent experimental activity against the *M. avium* complex. However, this experimental activity was later shown to be limited [84] and could not be clinically confirmed for the treatment of *M. avium* bacteremia in acquired immunodeficiency syndrome patients [85, 86].

With the emergence of MDR-TB, the interest in clofazimine was once more renewed. Although not scientifically proven to be active in human TB, clofazimine is among the drugs being considered among group 5 drugs for the treatment of MDR-/XDR-TB [68]. More recently, clofazimine has been used with great success in combined drug regimens of 9–12 months' duration for the treatment of MDR-TB [87–90]. As clofazimine contributed significant bactericidal and treatment-shortening activity in mouse models of both drug-susceptible and drug-resistant TB [91, 92], there is growing body of evidence supporting the inclusion of CFZ in drug regimens for the treatment of MDR-TB as well as drug-susceptible TB.

7.6   Immunization and Vaccines

It is common knowledge that the host resistance to tuberculosis is controlled by the cellular immunity which is driven by macrophages and T lymphocytes. For example, an effective immune system is crucial to contain latent infection with *M.tb*. Enhancing the effector mechanisms of these immune cells is the objective of vaccines to protect the host for getting infected by *M.tb* and host-directed therapies to reinforce the immune status and improve the effectiveness of antimicrobial treatment.

7.6.1   Vaccines

Although conferring good protection against miliary and meningeal tuberculosis in children, the only registered vaccine against tuberculosis, the Bacillus Calmette-Guérin (BCG) confers irregular and limited protection against pulmonary tuberculosis in all age groups [93]. For this very reason, numerous research groups did and do try to develop an improved vaccine against tuberculosis [94].

Given the advances in immunology and molecular biology since BCG was developed in the 1920s, safer and more elaborated vaccine strategies have been designed. These include, first, live recombinant BCG or other genetically modified mycobacteria often overexpressing dominant tuberculosis antigens that could be safer and/or more efficacious than BCG, thus replace it. They include also attenuated virus vectors, especially pox virus or adenovirus, genetically modified to express dominant tuberculosis antigen. An aim of these recombinant viral vectors is booster BCG vaccination. A third strategy is focusing, not on living vaccines, but on dominant tuberculosis proteins and adjuvants to booster specific immunity. As of yet, such strategies have not been successful. For example, the attenuated modified vaccinia Ankara, MVA85A, expressing the antigen 85 of *M.tb* failed to booster the effect of BCG vaccination [95, 96]; and the trial of the recombinant BCG vaccine (AERAS-422) overexpressing tuberculosis antigens and perfringolysin has to be stopped for safety reasons [94]. Even though current expectations in the tuberculosis vaccine development are not yet fulfilled, "strength lies in tenacity" as claimed by Stephan Kaufmann [97].

7.6.2 Host-Directed Therapies

Host-directed therapy is an immunotherapeutic approach which aims at eliminating *M.tb* by targeting the host [98, 99]. For a successful approach, diverse agents are used to regulate the immune response, through either the reduction of the tissue-damaging inflammation or the augmentation of the protective immune responses, for example, in patients with multidrug-resistant tuberculosis.

For the reduction of inflammatory response, analgesic or anti-inflammatory drugs such as ibuprofen, corticosteroids, TNF blockers, and leukotriene inhibitors are on the frontline. The phosphodiesterase inhibitors cilostazol and sildenafil have shown promise in animal models.

For the augmentation of the protective immune response, host-directed therapies include the use of immunomodulatory drugs that have the potential to enhance immune responses and need assessment for their usefulness as adjunct therapies with antituberculosis drugs to improve cure rates for MDR disease, shorten duration of therapy, and prevent recurrence. These include mycobacterial antigens or whole-cell inactivated environmental mycobacteria and cytokines (interleukin 2, interleukin 7, and interferon γ).

Host-directed therapy may aim also at enhancing antimicrobial mechanisms by autophagy inducers which would deliver potentially harmful cytosolic macromolecules and organelles to lysosomes for *M.tb* degradation, by protein kinase inhibitors, by cathelicidin inducers, by metformin, and by high-dose immunoglobulins. Another way to enhance antimicrobial activity is through efflux pump inhibitors such as verapamil and reserpine which would increase the drug exposure in case of drug susceptibility or partly restore susceptibility to antituberculosis drugs in case of drug resistance.

References

1. WHO. Global tuberculosis report. Geneva, Switzerland; 2014.
2. Zumla A, Chakaya J, Centis R, D'Ambrosio L, Mwaba P, Bates M, et al. Tuberculosis treatment and management--an update on treatment regimens, trials, new drugs, and adjunct therapies. Lancet Respir Med. 2015;3(3):220–34.
3. Pethe K, Bifani P, Jang J, Kang S, Park S, Ahn S, et al. Discovery of Q203, a potent clinical candidate for the treatment of tuberculosis. Nat Med. 2013;19(9):1157–60.
4. Andries K, Verhasselt P, Guillemont J, Gohlmann HW, Neefs JM, Winkler H, et al. A diarylquinoline drug active on the ATP synthase of Mycobacterium tuberculosis. Science. 2005; 307(5707):223–7.
5. Makarov V, Manina G, Mikusova K, Mollmann U, Ryabova O, Saint-Joanis B, et al. Benzothiazinones kill Mycobacterium tuberculosis by blocking arabinan synthesis. Science. 2009;324(5928):801–4.
6. Makarov V, Lechartier B, Zhang M, Neres J, van der Sar AM, Raadsen SA, et al. Towards a new combination therapy for tuberculosis with next generation benzothiazinones. EMBO Mol Med. 2014;6(3):372–83.
7. FDA U. 2012 [updated 15 March 2015]. December 31, 2012 [United States Food and Drug Administration]. Available from: http://www.fda.gov/NewsEvents/Newsroom/Press Announcements/ucm333695.htm.
8. FDA U. Briefing Package: NDA 204–384. 2012.
9. EMA. EMA/794261/2013. 2013;20 December 2013.
10. WHO. The use of bedaquiline in the treatment of multidrug-resistant tuberculosis. Interim policy guidance. Geneva; 2013.
11. Andries K, Gevers T, Lounis N. Bactericidal potencies of new regimens are not predictive of their sterilizing potencies in a murine model of tuberculosis. Antimicrob Agents Chemother. 2010;54(11):4540–4.
12. Ibrahim M, Andries K, Lounis N, Chauffour A, Truffot-Pernot C, Jarlier V, et al. Synergistic activity of R207910 combined with pyrazinamide against murine tuberculosis. Antimicrob Agents Chemother. 2007;51(3):1011–5.
13. Ibrahim M, Truffot-Pernot C, Andries K, Jarlier V, Veziris N. Sterilizing activity of R207910 (TMC207)-containing regimens in the murine model of tuberculosis. Am J Respir Crit Care Med. 2009;180(6):553–7.

14. Lounis N, Gevers T, Van Den Berg J, Andries K. Impact of the interaction of R207910 with rifampin on the treatment of tuberculosis studied in the mouse model. Antimicrob Agents Chemother. 2008;52(10):3568–72.

15. Lounis N, Veziris N, Chauffour A, Truffot-Pernot C, Andries K, Jarlier V. Combinations of R207910 with drugs used to treat multidrug-resistant tuberculosis have the potential to shorten treatment duration. Antimicrob Agents Chemother. 2006;50(11): 3543–7.

16. Rouan MC, Lounis N, Gevers T, Dillen L, Gilissen R, Raoof A, et al. Pharmacokinetics and pharmacodynamics of TMC207 and its N-desmethyl metabolite in a murine model of tuberculosis. Antimicrob Agents Chemother. 2012;56(3):1444–51.

17. Veziris N, Ibrahim M, Lounis N, Andries K, Jarlier V. Sterilizing activity of second-line regimens containing TMC207 in a murine model of tuberculosis. PLoS One. 2011;6(3), e17556.

18. Rustomjee R, Diacon AH, Allen J, Venter A, Reddy C, Patientia RF, et al. Early bactericidal activity and pharmacokinetics of the diarylquinoline TMC207 in treatment of pulmonary tuberculosis. Antimicrob Agents Chemother. 2008;52(8):2831–5.

19. Diacon AH, Dawson R, von Groote-Bidlingmaier F, Symons G, Venter A, Donald PR, et al. 14-day bactericidal activity of PA-824, bedaquiline, pyrazinamide, and moxifloxacin combinations: a randomised trial. Lancet. 2012;380(9846):986–93.

20. Diacon AH, Dawson R, von Groote-Bidlingmaier F, Symons G, Venter A, Donald PR, et al. Bactericidal activity of pyrazinamide and clofazimine alone and in combinations with pretomanid and bedaquiline. Am J Respir Crit Care Med. 2015;191(8):943–53.

21. Diacon AH, Pym A, Grobusch M, Patientia R, Rustomjee R, Page-Shipp L, et al. The diarylquinoline TMC207 for multidrug-resistant tuberculosis. N Engl J Med. 2009;360(23):2397–405.

22. Diacon AH, Donald PR, Pym A, Grobusch M, Patientia RF, Mahanyele R, et al. Randomized pilot trial of eight weeks of bedaquiline (TMC207) treatment for multidrug-resistant tuberculosis: long-term outcome, tolerability, and effect on emergence of drug resistance. Antimicrob Agents Chemother. 2012;56(6):3271–6.

23. Diacon AH, Pym A, Grobusch MP, de los Rios JM, Gotuzzo E, Vasilyeva I, et al. Multidrug-resistant tuberculosis and culture conversion with bedaquiline. N Engl J Med. 2014;371(8): 723–32.

24. Guglielmetti L, Le Du D, Jachym M, Henry B, Martin D, Caumes E, et al. Compassionate use of bedaquiline for the treatment of

multidrug-resistant and extensively drug-resistant tuberculosis: interim analysis of a French cohort. Clin Infect Dis. 2015;60(2): 188–94.

25. Matsumoto M, Hashizume H, Tomishige T, Kawasaki M, Tsubouchi H, Sasaki H, et al. OPC-67683, a nitro-dihydro-imidazooxazole derivative with promising action against tuberculosis in vitro and in mice. PLoS Med. 2006;3(11), e466.

26. Diacon AH, Dawson R, Hanekom M, Narunsky K, Venter A, Hittel N, et al. Early bactericidal activity of delamanid (OPC-67683) in smear-positive pulmonary tuberculosis patients. Int J Tuberc Lung Dis. 2011;15(7):949–54.

27. Gler MT, Skripconoka V, Sanchez-Garavito E, Xiao H, Cabrera-Rivero JL, Vargas-Vasquez DE, et al. Delamanid for multidrug-resistant pulmonary tuberculosis. N Engl J Med. 2012;366(23):2151–60.

28. Gupta R, Geiter LJ, Wells CD, Gao M, Cirule A, Xiao H. Delamanid for extensively drug-resistant tuberculosis. N Engl J Med. 2015;373(3):291–2.

29. Stover CK, Warrener P, VanDevanter DR, Sherman DR, Arain TM, Langhorne MH, et al. A small-molecule nitroimidazopyran drug candidate for the treatment of tuberculosis. Nature. 2000;405(6789):962–6.

30. Ginsberg AM, Laurenzi MW, Rouse DJ, Whitney KD, Spigelman MK. Safety, tolerability, and pharmacokinetics of PA-824 in healthy subjects. Antimicrob Agents Chemother. 2009;53(9): 3720–5.

31. Tyagi S, Nuermberger E, Yoshimatsu T, Williams K, Rosenthal I, Lounis N, et al. Bactericidal activity of the nitroimidazopyran PA-824 in a murine model of tuberculosis. Antimicrob Agents Chemother. 2005;49(6):2289–93.

32. Nuermberger E, Tyagi S, Tasneen R, Williams KN, Almeida D, Rosenthal I, et al. Powerful bactericidal and sterilizing activity of a regimen containing PA-824, moxifloxacin, and pyrazinamide in a murine model of tuberculosis. Antimicrob Agents Chemother. 2008;52(4):1522–4.

33. Dawson R, Diacon AH, Everitt D, van Niekerk C, Donald PR, Burger DA, et al. Efficiency and safety of the combination of moxifloxacin, pretomanid (PA-824), and pyrazinamide during the first 8 weeks of antituberculosis treatment: a phase 2b, open-label, partly randomised trial in patients with drug-susceptible or drug-resistant pulmonary tuberculosis. Lancet. 2015;385(9979): 1738–47.

34. Kmentova I, Sutherland HS, Palmer BD, Blaser A, Franzblau SG, Wan B, et al. Synthesis and structure-activity relationships of aza- and diazabiphenyl analogues of the antitubercular drug (6S)-2-nitro-6-{[4-(trifluoromethoxy)benzyl]oxy}-6,7-dihydro-5H-imidazo[2,1-b][1, 3]oxazine (PA-824). J Med Chem. 2010;53(23):8421–39.

35. Upton AM, Cho S, Yang TJ, Kim Y, Wang Y, Lu Y, et al. In vitro and in vivo activities of the nitroimidazole TBA-354 against Mycobacterium tuberculosis. Antimicrob Agents Chemother. 2015;59(1):136–44.

36. Tasneen R, Williams K, Amoabeng O, Minkowski A, Mdluli KE, Upton AM, et al. Contribution of the nitroimidazoles PA-824 and TBA-354 to the activity of novel regimens in murine models of tuberculosis. Antimicrob Agents Chemother. 2015;59(1): 129–35.

37. Barbachyn MR, Hutchinson DK, Brickner SJ, Cynamon MH, Kilburn JO, Klemens SP, et al. Identification of a novel oxazolidinone (U-100480) with potent antimycobacterial activity. J Med Chem. 1996;39(3):680–5.

38. Shaw KJ, Barbachyn MR. The oxazolidinones: past, present, and future. Ann N Y Acad Sci. 2011;1241:48–70.

39. Stalker DJ, Jungbluth GL. Clinical pharmacokinetics of linezolid, a novel oxazolidinone antibacterial. Clin Pharmacokinet. 2003;42(13):1129–40.

40. Huang TS, Liu YC, Sy CL, Chen YS, Tu HZ, Chen BC. In vitro activities of linezolid against clinical isolates of Mycobacterium tuberculosis complex isolated in Taiwan over 10 years. Antimicrob Agents Chemother. 2008;52(6):2226–7.

41. Dietze R, Hadad DJ, McGee B, Molino LP, Maciel EL, Peloquin CA, et al. Early and extended early bactericidal activity of linezolid in pulmonary tuberculosis. Am J Respir Crit Care Med. 2008;178(11):1180–5.

42. McKee EE, Ferguson M, Bentley AT, Marks TA. Inhibition of mammalian mitochondrial protein synthesis by oxazolidinones. Antimicrob Agents Chemother. 2006;50(6):2042–9.

43. Migliori GB, Eker B, Richardson MD, Sotgiu G, Zellweger JP, Skrahina A, et al. A retrospective TBNET assessment of linezolid safety, tolerability and efficacy in multidrug-resistant tuberculosis. Eur Respir J. 2009;34(2):387–93.

44. Yew WW, Chau CH, Wen KH. Linezolid in the treatment of 'difficult' multidrug-resistant tuberculosis. Int J Tuberc Lung Dis. 2008;12(3):345–6.

45. Lee M, Cho SN, Barry 3rd CE, Song T, Kim Y, Jeong I. Linezolid for XDR-TB – final study outcomes. N Engl J Med. 2015;373(3):290–1.
46. Lee M, Lee J, Carroll MW, Choi H, Min S, Song T, et al. Linezolid for treatment of chronic extensively drug-resistant tuberculosis. N Engl J Med. 2012;367(16):1508–18.
47. Cox H, Ford N. Linezolid for the treatment of complicated drug-resistant tuberculosis: a systematic review and meta-analysis. Int J Tuberc Lung Dis. 2012;16(4):447–54.
48. Chang KC, Yew WW, Cheung SW, Leung CC, Tam CM, Chau CH, et al. Can intermittent dosing optimize prolonged linezolid treatment of difficult multidrug-resistant tuberculosis? Antimicrob Agents Chemother. 2013;57(7):3445–9.
49. Williams KN, Stover CK, Zhu T, Tasneen R, Tyagi S, Grosset JH, et al. Promising antituberculosis activity of the oxazolidinone PNU-100480 relative to that of linezolid in a murine model. Antimicrob Agents Chemother. 2009;53(4):1314–9.
50. Williams KN, Brickner SJ, Stover CK, Zhu T, Ogden A, Tasneen R, et al. Addition of PNU-100480 to first-line drugs shortens the time needed to cure murine tuberculosis. Am J Respir Crit Care Med. 2009;180(4):371–6.
51. Wallis RS, Jakubiec W, Mitton-Fry M, Ladutko L, Campbell S, Paige D, et al. Rapid evaluation in whole blood culture of regimens for XDR-TB containing PNU-100480 (sutezolid), TMC207, PA-824, SQ109, and pyrazinamide. PLoS One. 2012;7(1), e30479.
52. Wallis RS, Dawson R, Friedrich SO, Venter A, Paige D, Zhu T, et al. Mycobactericidal activity of sutezolid (PNU-100480) in sputum (EBA) and blood (WBA) of patients with pulmonary tuberculosis. PLoS One. 2014;9(4), e94462.
53. Vera-Cabrera L, Gonzalez E, Rendon A, Ocampo-Candiani J, Welsh O, Velazquez-Moreno VM, et al. In vitro activities of DA-7157 and DA-7218 against Mycobacterium tuberculosis and Nocardia brasiliensis. Antimicrob Agents Chemother. 2006;50(9):3170–2.
54. Urbina O, Ferrandez O, Espona M, Salas E, Ferrandez I, Grau S. Potential role of tedizolid phosphate in the treatment of acute bacterial skin infections. Drug Des Devel Ther. 2013;7:243–65.
55. Prokocimer P, De Anda C, Fang E, Mehra P, Das A. Tedizolid phosphate vs linezolid for treatment of acute bacterial skin and skin structure infections: the ESTABLISH-1 randomized trial. JAMA. 2013;309(6):559–69.
56. Moran GJ, Fang E, Corey GR, Das AF, De Anda C, Prokocimer P. Tedizolid for 6 days versus linezolid for 10 days for acute bacterial skin and skin-structure infections (ESTABLISH-2): a

randomised, double-blind, phase 3, non-inferiority trial. Lancet Infect Dis. 2014;14(8):696–705.

57. Johnson JL, Hadad DJ, Boom WH, Daley CL, Peloquin CA, Eisenach KD, Jankus DD, Debanne SM, Charlebois ED, Maciel E, Palaci M, Dietze R. Early and extended early bactericidal activity of levofloxacin, gatifloxacin and moxifloxacin in pulmonary tuberculosis. Int J Tuberc Lung Dis. 2006;10(6):605–12.

58. Nuermberger EL, Yoshimatsu T, Tyagi S, O'Brien RJ, Vernon AN, Chaisson RE, Bishai WR, Grosset JH. Moxifloxacin-containing regimen greatly reduces time to culture conversion in murine tuberculosis. Am J Respir Crit Care Med. 2004;169(3):421–6.

59. Ji B, Lounis N, Maslo C, Truffot-Pernot C, Bonnafous P, Grosset J. In vitro and in vivo activities of moxifloxacin and clinafloxacin against Mycobacterium tuberculosis. Antimicrob Agents Chemother. 1998;42(8):2066–9.

60. Nuermberger EL, Yoshimatsu T, Tyagi S, O'Brien RJ, Vernon AN, Chaisson RE, et al. Moxifloxacin-containing regimen greatly reduces time to culture conversion in murine tuberculosis. Am J Respir Crit Care Med. 2004;169(3):421–6.

61. Pletz MW, De Roux A, Roth A, Neumann KH, Mauch H, Lode H. Early bactericidal activity of moxifloxacin in treatment of pulmonary tuberculosis: a prospective, randomized study. Antimicrob Agents Chemother. 2004;48(3):780–2.

62. Dorman SE, Johnson JL, Goldberg S, Muzanye G, Padayatchi N, Bozeman L, et al. Substitution of moxifloxacin for isoniazid during intensive phase treatment of pulmonary tuberculosis. Am J Respir Crit Care Med. 2009;180(3):273–80.

63. Conde MB, Efron A, Loredo C, De Souza GR, Graca NP, Cezar MC, et al. Moxifloxacin versus ethambutol in the initial treatment of tuberculosis: a double-blind, randomised, controlled phase II trial. Lancet. 2009;373(9670):1183–9.

64. Rustomjee R, Lienhardt C, Kanyok T, Davies GR, Levin J, Mthiyane T, et al. A Phase II study of the sterilising activities of ofloxacin, gatifloxacin and moxifloxacin in pulmonary tuberculosis. Int J Tuberc Lung Dis. 2008;12(2):128–38.

65. Merle CS, Fielding K, Sow OB, Gninafon M, Lo MB, Mthiyane T, et al. A four-month gatifloxacin-containing regimen for treating tuberculosis. N Engl J Med. 2014;371(17):1588–98.

66. Gillespie SH, Crook AM, McHugh TD, Mendel CM, Meredith SK, Murray SR, et al. Four-month moxifloxacin-based regimens for drug-sensitive tuberculosis. N Engl J Med. 2014;371(17):1577–87.

67. Jindani A, Harrison TS, Nunn AJ, Phillips PP, Churchyard GJ, Charalambous S, et al. High-dose rifapentine with moxifloxacin for pulmonary tuberculosis. N Engl J Med. 2014;371(17):1599–608.
68. WHO. Companion handbook to the WHO guidelines for the programmatic management of drug-resistant tuberculosis. Geneva; 2014.
69. Walsh C. Antibiotics: actions, origins, resistance. Walsh C, editor. Washington, DC: ASM Press; 2003. p. 23–49.
70. Hamad B. The antibiotics market. Nat Rev Drug Discov. 2010;9(9):675–6.
71. Hugonnet JE, Blanchard JS. Irreversible inhibition of the Mycobacterium tuberculosis beta-lactamase by clavulanate. Biochemistry. 2007;46(43):11998–2004.
72. Hugonnet JE, Tremblay LW, Boshoff HI, Barry 3rd CE, Blanchard JS. Meropenem-clavulanate is effective against extensively drug-resistant Mycobacterium tuberculosis. Science. 2009;323(5918):1215–8.
73. Lavollay M, Arthur M, Fourgeaud M, Dubost L, Marie A, Veziris N, et al. The peptidoglycan of stationary-phase Mycobacterium tuberculosis predominantly contains cross-links generated by L,D-transpeptidation. J Bacteriol. 2008; 190(12):4360–6.
74. Gupta R, Lavollay M, Mainardi JL, Arthur M, Bishai WR, Lamichhane G. The Mycobacterium tuberculosis protein LdtMt2 is a nonclassical transpeptidase required for virulence and resistance to amoxicillin. Nat Med. 2010;16(4):466–9.
75. Goffin C, Ghuysen JM. Biochemistry and comparative genomics of SxxK superfamily acyltransferases offer a clue to the mycobacterial paradox: presence of penicillin-susceptible target proteins versus lack of efficiency of penicillin as therapeutic agent. Microbiol Mol Biol Rev. 2002;66(4):702–38.
76. Horita Y, Maeda S, Kazumi Y, Doi N. In vitro susceptibility of Mycobacterium tuberculosis isolates to an oral carbapenem alone or in combination with beta-lactamase inhibitors. Antimicrob Agents Chemother. 2014;58(11):7010–4.
77. Hazra S, Xu H, Blanchard JS. Tebipenem, a new carbapenem antibiotic, is a slow substrate that inhibits the beta-lactamase from Mycobacterium tuberculosis. Biochemistry. 2014;53(22): 3671–8.
78. Dhar N, Dubee V, Ballell L, Cuinet G, Hugonnet JE, Signorino-Gelo F, et al. Rapid cytolysis of Mycobacterium tuberculosis by faropenem, an orally bioavailable beta-lactam antibiotic. Antimicrob Agents Chemother. 2015;59(2):1308–19.

79. Kaushik A, Makkar N, Pandey P, Parrish N, Singh U, Lamichhane G. Carbapenems and rifampicin exhibit synergy against Mycobacterium tuberculosis and Mycobacterium abscessus. Antimicrob Agents Chemother. 2015;59(10):6561–7.

80. Keener AB. Oldie but goodie: repurposing penicillin for tuberculosis. Nat Med. 2014;20(9):976–8.

81. Dooley KE, Bliven-Sizemore EE, Weiner M, Lu Y, Nuermberger EL, Hubbard WC, et al. Safety and pharmacokinetics of escalating daily doses of the antituberculosis drug rifapentine in healthy volunteers. Clin Pharmacol Ther. 2012;91(5):881–8.

82. Dorman SE, Savic RM, Goldberg S, Stout JE, Schluger N, Muzanyi G, et al. Daily rifapentine for treatment of pulmonary tuberculosis. A randomized, dose-ranging trial. Am J Respir Crit Care Med. 2015;191(3):333–43.

83. Barry VC, Conalty ML. The antimycobacterial activity of B 663. Lepr Rev. 1965;36:3–7.

84. Lounis N, Gevers T, Van den Berg J, Vranckx L, Andries K. ATP synthase inhibition of Mycobacterium avium is not bactericidal. Antimicrob Agents Chemother. 2009;53(11):4927–9.

85. Chaisson RE, Keiser P, Pierce M, Fessel WJ, Ruskin J, Lahart C, et al. Clarithromycin and ethambutol with or without clofazimine for the treatment of bacteremic Mycobacterium avium complex disease in patients with HIV infection. AIDS. 1997;11(3):311–7.

86. Shafran SD, Singer J, Zarowny DP, Phillips P, Salit I, Walmsley SL, et al. A comparison of two regimens for the treatment of Mycobacterium avium complex bacteremia in AIDS: rifabutin, ethambutol, and clarithromycin versus rifampin, ethambutol, clofazimine, and ciprofloxacin. Canadian HIV Trials Network Protocol 010 Study Group. N Engl J Med. 1996;335(6):377–83.

87. Aung KJ, Van Deun A, Declercq E, Sarker MR, Das PK, Hossain MA, et al. Successful '9-month Bangladesh regimen' for multidrug-resistant tuberculosis among over 500 consecutive patients. Int J Tuberc Lung Dis. 2014;18(10):1180–7.

88. Kuaban C, Noeske J, Rieder HL, Ait-Khaled N, Abena Foe JL, Trebucq A. High effectiveness of a 12-month regimen for MDR-TB patients in Cameroon. Int J Tuberc Lung Dis. 2015;19(5):517–24.

89. Tang S, Yao L, Hao X, Liu Y, Zeng L, Liu G, et al. Clofazimine for the treatment of multidrug-resistant tuberculosis: prospective, multicenter, randomized controlled study in China. Clin Infect Dis. 2015;60(9):1361–7.

90. Van Deun A, Maug AK, Salim MA, Das PK, Sarker MR, Daru P, et al. Short, highly effective, and inexpensive standardized

treatment of multidrug-resistant tuberculosis. Am J Respir Crit Care Med. 2010;182(5):684–92.

91. Grosset JH, Tyagi S, Almeida DV, Converse PJ, Li SY, Ammerman NC, et al. Assessment of clofazimine activity in a second-line regimen for tuberculosis in mice. Am J Respir Crit Care Med. 2013;188(5):608–12.

92. Tyagi S, Ammerman NC, Li SY, Adamson J, Converse PJ, Swanson RV, et al. Clofazimine shortens the duration of the first-line treatment regimen for experimental chemotherapy of tuberculosis. Proc Natl Acad Sci U S A. 2015;112(3):869–74.

93. Mangtani P, Abubakar I, Ariti C, Beynon R, Pimpin L, Fine PE, et al. Protection by BCG vaccine against tuberculosis: a systematic review of randomized controlled trials. Clin Infect Dis. 2014;58(4):470–80.

94. Hokey DA, Ginsberg A. The current state of tuberculosis vaccines. Human Vaccines Immunother. 2013;9(10):2142–6.

95. Tameris M, Geldenhuys H, Luabeya AK, Smit E, Hughes JE, Vermaak S, et al. The candidate TB vaccine, MVA85A, induces highly durable Th1 responses. PLoS One. 2014;9(2), e87340.

96. Tameris MD, Hatherill M, Landry BS, Scriba TJ, Snowden MA, Lockhart S, et al. Safety and efficacy of MVA85A, a new tuberculosis vaccine, in infants previously vaccinated with BCG: a randomised, placebo-controlled phase 2b trial. Lancet. 2013;381(9871):1021–8.

97. Kaufmann SH. Tuberculosis vaccine development: strength lies in tenacity. Trends Immunol. 2012;33(7):373–9.

98. Kaufmann SH, Lange C, Rao M, Balaji KN, Lotze M, Schito M, et al. Progress in tuberculosis vaccine development and host-directed therapies--a state of the art review. Lancet Respir Med. 2014;2(4):301–20.

99. Wallis RS, Hafner R. Advancing host-directed therapy for tuberculosis. Nat Rev Immunol. 2015;15(4):255–63.

Chapter 8
Conclusions and Future Directions

Richard E. Chaisson and Jacques H. Grosset

In the century between the discovery of the tubercle bacillus by Koch and the development of the current all oral, short-course chemotherapy that cures tuberculosis in just 6 months, the world witnessed extraordinary biomedical progress that seemingly tamed a once-fearsome killer. Regrettably, the biomedical community declared a premature end to the hostilities, assumed that tuberculosis was a solved problem, and moved on to other challenges. Tuberculosis control was relegated to public health departments, and tuberculosis research and training essentially evaporated. While great progress was made in controlling tuberculosis in wealthy countries, the global burden of the disease was never diminished, and the advent of the HIV epidemic and the emergence of drug-resistant disease ushered in a new global crisis that continues today. A great tragedy in the exodus of tuberculosis research and teaching in academic centers was a

R.E. Chaisson
Department of Medicine, Epidemiology, and International Health, Johns Hopkins University, Baltimore, MD, USA

J.H. Grosset (✉)
Department of Medicine, Johns Hopkins University School of Medicine, 1550 Orleans St, Rm 105, Baltimore, MD 21231, USA
e-mail: jgrosse4@jhmi.edu

J.H. Grosset, R.E. Chaisson (eds.), *Handbook of Tuberculosis*,   219
DOI 10.1007/978-3-319-26273-4_8,
© Springer International Publishing Switzerland 2017

loss of interest in innovation, discovery, and improvement to the tools available to contain the disease. Only in recent years has the global public health community recognized the importance of continually seeking to find new tools and strategies to combat the disease.

The World Health Organization has created the End TB Strategy as an aspiration for the next 20 years of tuberculosis control, with the ambitious targets of a 90 % reduction in tuberculosis incidence, 95 % reduction in tuberculosis deaths, and an end to catastrophic personal costs to individuals and families affected by tuberculosis [1]. Such enormous decreases in the burden of tuberculosis are clearly not feasible given current resources, health systems, and tools, however, and the WHO acknowledges the need for developing new tools and new public health strategies for ending the tuberculosis epidemic [2]. Current rates of decline in tuberculosis incidence are between 1 % and 2 % per year, and achieving the 90 % target requires >15 % reductions annually for the next 20 years. Accelerating the implementation of currently available tools would increase the rate of decline to up to 10 % per year according to mathematical modeling, yet we would still fall short. Thus, the success of the End TB Strategy relies on developing a new arsenal of diagnostics, biomarkers, drugs to treat and prevent tuberculosis, and a highly effective vaccine. In addition, implementation science, the process of investigating the most effective methods for delivering interventions with proved efficacy to the populations that will benefit from them, will be an essential element of future tuberculosis research. Public health strategies for controlling tuberculosis have been based solely on the model of identifying and treating cases of disease since the 1970s, in the mistaken belief that case finding and prescribing the adequate treatment were all that was necessary to reduce incidence. Scant attention has been paid to preventing tuberculosis, even in the highest-risk populations with latent infection, such as young children, household contacts, and people with HIV infection. Epidemic modeling now clearly demonstrates that attacking the reservoir of latent infections that give rise to future cases is required if tuberculosis is to be contained. Ultimately, a new vaccine that prevents infectious cases from occurring will be the true End TB strategy. Until such a preventative is developed, however, huge improvements in implementing all of the currently available *and* newly developed tools to detect, treat, and prevent transmission of the organism and to treat latent tuberculosis will be necessary to approach the bold targets set by the WHO.

This book has provided a basic yet comprehensive overview of tuberculosis, including its history, epidemiology, pathogenesis, diagnosis, treatment, and prevention. Our last chapter, Emerging Therapies, offered a snapshot of some of the exciting work currently underway to discover and develop more effective therapeutic agents. The last chapter of tuberculosis, however, will not be written until numerous innovations, discoveries, and breakthroughs are achieved and brought to the people and communities who most desperately need them. Whether it be in the laboratory, the classroom, the clinic, the hospital, the community, or public health agencies, we encourage you to contribute to this essential task.

References

1. Upkelar M, Weill D, Lonnroth K, et al. WHO's new end TB strategy. Lancet. 2015;385:1799–801.
2. Dye C, Glaziou P, Floyd K, Raviglione MC. Prospects for tuberculosis elimination. Annu Rev Public Health. 2013;34:271–86.

Printed in the United States
By Bookmasters